ATLAS OF
FORENSIC
PATHOLOGY

*"Those who have dissected or inspected many bodies have at least
learned to doubt, while those who are ignorant of anatomy and do not
take the trouble to attend to it, are in no doubt at all."*

—Giovanni Morgagni
The Father of Morbid Anatomy

ATLAS OF FORENSIC PATHOLOGY

B Suresh Kumar Shetty MBBS MD PGCTM
Professor and Head

Prateek Rastogi MBBS MD PGDMLE PGDCFS
Dip Cyber Law PGCMNCPA PGCTM
Associate Professor

Jagadish Rao Padubidri MBBS MD DNB
PGDCFS PGCTM Dip Cyber Law MNAMS
Associate Professor

Tanuj Kanchan MBBS DFM MD
Associate Professor

YP Raghavendra Babu MBBS MD
Associate Professor

Department of Forensic Medicine and Toxicology
Kasturba Medical College
(A constituent college of Manipal University)
Mangalore, Karnataka, India

Forewords

K Ramnarayan
G Pradeep Kumar
DS Badkur

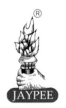

JAYPEE

JAYPEE BROTHERS MEDICAL PUBLISHERS (P) LTD
New Delhi • London • Philadelphia • Panama

Jaypee Brothers Medical Publishers (P) Ltd

Headquarters

Jaypee Brothers Medical Publishers (P) Ltd
4838/24, Ansari Road, Daryaganj
New Delhi 110 002, India
Phone: +91-11-43574357
Fax: +91-11-43574314
Email: jaypee@jaypeebrothers.com

Overseas Offices

J.P. Medical Ltd
83 Victoria Street, London
SW1H 0HW (UK)
Phone: +44-2031708910
Fax: +02-03-0086180
Email: info@jpmedpub.com

Jaypee Medical Inc
The Bourse
111 South Independence Mall East
Suite 835, Philadelphia, PA 19106, USA
Phone: +1 267-519-9789
Email: jpmed.us@gmail.com

Jaypee Brothers Medical Publishers (P) Ltd
Bhotahity, Kathmandu, Nepal
Phone: +977-9741283608
Email: kathmandu@jaypeebrothers.com

Jaypee-Highlights Medical Publishers Inc
City of Knowledge, Bld. 237, Clayton
Panama City, Panama
Phone: +1 507-301-0496
Fax: +1 507-301-0499
Email: cservice@jphmedical.com

Jaypee Brothers Medical Publishers (P) Ltd
17/1-B Babar Road, Block-B, Shaymali
Mohammadpur, Dhaka-1207
Bangladesh
Mobile: +08801912003485
Email: jaypeedhaka@gmail.com

Website: www.jaypeebrothers.com
Website: www.jaypeedigital.com

Inquiries for bulk sales may be solicited at: jaypee@jaypeebrothers.com

Atlas of Forensic Pathology

First Edition: **2014**

ISBN 978-93-5090-468-8

Printed at: Samrat Offset Pvt. Ltd.

Foreword

I am delighted to write this message for the *Atlas of Forensic Pathology* authored by Dr B Suresh Kumar Shetty, Dr Prateek Rastogi, Dr Tanuj Kanchan, Dr Jagadish Rao Padubidri and Dr YP Raghavendra Babu. Pictures are invaluable in capturing the interest of the reader. The clarity of the photographs and the full spectrum of the lesions provide a learning opportunity for the neophyte as well as to the specialist. The authors are not only well qualified, but also they have a commitment and experience in teaching Forensic Medicine for several years, in addition to having commendable research publications. Let me extend my warmest felicitations to all the authors and wish them many more publications in the years to come.

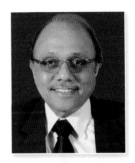

K Ramnarayan MBBS MD
Vice-Chancellor
Manipal University
Manipal, Karnataka, India

Foreword

Healthcare and law enforcement professionals that include the police and the legal fraternity have the unique opportunity to make a difference in the lives of the public by providing justice to the victims of assault, be it trauma, sexual or otherwise. It is the duty of the forensic pathologist to diagnose the various objectives of a medicolegal autopsy, assimilate the medical evidence, and present it in a manner that could be clearly understood by the legal and judicial fraternity that would enable them to deliver justice. A forensic pathologist's job does not end with an autopsy, but foresee issues that could arise, weeks, months, years or even decades after the crime has occurred; hence, a complete understanding of the subject is very essential.

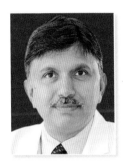

As forensic pathology has progressed over the century from less evidence based to more evidence based, so have the literature and textbooks have improved over the years. *Atlas of Forensic Pathology* is such an example of an accomplishment with numerous photographs, brief but adequate description that would enable the health care, legal and police professionals achieve their goals of providing justice to the society.

The authors have designed the atlas keeping in mind the practical requirements and the needs of the doctors practicing forensic medicine, the lawmakers, and the law enforcing agencies. Every segment of the forensic pathology requirements of the body has been kept in mind while designing the core content of this atlas. The pictures speak volumes of the emphasis on various practical aspects in the practice of the forensic medicine that has been dealt with excellently through illustrations. I would like to compliment the various contributors of this manual for their commitment and efforts to make the challenging practice of forensic medicine much easier.

This manual, though the authors claim to have designed for undergraduates and general practitioners, I strongly feel that it is a very useful book for the postgraduates pursuing MD in Forensic Medicine, police officers and to the legal fraternity.

I strongly recommend this book to be an integral part of learning the art and science of forensic medicine to both the undergraduates and postgraduates of forensic medicine. Not only students, every practitioner of forensic medicine should possess a copy of this manual for ready reference.

G Pradeep Kumar MD
Professor
Department of Forensic Medicine
Dean
Kasturba Medical College
Manipal University
Manipal, Karnataka, India

Foreword

The *Atlas of Forensic Pathology* written by Dr B Suresh Kumar Shetty and his team of forensic experts comprising of Dr Prateek Rastogi, Dr Tanuj Kanchan, Dr Jagadish Rao Padubidri and Dr YP Raghavendra Babu all Associate Professors in the Department of Forensic Medicine, Kasturba Medical College, Mangalore (Manipal University) is an "objective atlas" on this subject and this idea is in fact very much open to questions. The atlas presents a picture of intense subject like Forensic Medicine to a lucid one. On close observation, one may find that these observations, by the editors of this atlas are exceptional. Each individual picture in this atlas is apt 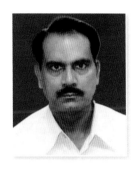 and is picked without any bend because the editors would not have selected them otherwise. Details in the form of captions turn out to contain great significance and relevance to the topics. The uncommon conditions made in the various visual inventories reveal things that usually remain invisible or difficult to see in one's career. In contrast to often propagandist tenor of books, this atlas shows a complex reality that lies beyond simplistic and blinding pictorial images.

At the best, I hope that this pluralistic representation can contribute more among the undergraduates, postgraduates, forensic experts, lawyers and police officials. This potent series of alternative copyright-free images can serve as an inspiring freely available tool, which can be used to answer critical questions which are apparently objective.

DS Badkur MBBS MD DFM LLB FIAFM
Former President
Indian Academy of Forensic Medicine

Preface

It is our pleasure to place before you the *Atlas of Forensic Pathology*, the maiden venture from Department of Forensic Medicine and Toxicology, Kasturba Medical College, (A constituent college of Manipal University), Mangalore, Karnataka, India. Forensic Pathology is one of the major portions of broad specialty of Forensic Medicine comprising mainly of traumatology and thanatology. This atlas has been designed to incorporate a wide range of pictures from topics such as postmortem changes, mechanical injuries, firearm injuries, thermal injuries, road traffic accidents, regional injuries, mechanical asphyxia, transportation injuries, etc.

We hope that it will be useful to practitioners of forensic medicine, casualty medical officers, police persons, undergraduate and postgraduate students of forensic medicine.

B Suresh Kumar Shetty
Prateek Rastogi
Tanuj Kanchan
Jagadish Rao Padubidri
YP Raghavendra Babu

Acknowledgments

We are grateful to Dr Ramdas M Pai, Chancellor, Manipal University; Dr HS Ballal, Pro-Chancellor, Manipal University; Dr K Ramnarayan, Vice-Chancellor, Manipal University; Dr Surendra V Shetty, Pro Vice-Chancellor, Manipal University (Mangalore Campus), and Dr M Venkatraya Prabhu, Dean, Kasturba Medical College (KMC) (a constituent college of Manipal University), Mangalore, for their constant encouragement and guidance.

Dr G Pradeep Kumar, Professor and Dean, Kasturba Medical College, Manipal, and Dr Vikram Palimar, Professor and Head, Department of Forensic Medicine, Kasturba Medical College, Manipal, for their enriching support.

We like to pen down special thanks to former Heads of our department Late Dr KM Saralaya and Late Dr Anand Menon, for their motivating words in coming out with this book.

We wish to thank Professors and Heads of Department of Forensic Medicine of all neighboring colleges in and around Mangalore, for their valuable feedback and suggestions.

We wish to express our solemn sentiments and sincere thanks to all our colleagues of KMC, Manipal, friends, undergraduates and postgraduate students, and non-teaching staffs of KMC, Mangalore and Manipal.

We wholeheartedly thank Shri Jitendar P Vij (Group Chairman), Mr Ankit Vij (Managing Director) and Mr Tarun Duneja (Director-Publishing) of M/s Jaypee Brothers Medical Publishers (P) Ltd, New Delhi, India, for publishing the book in the same format as wanted well in time.

We acknowledge the wonderful work done by Ms Sunita Katla (Publishing Manager), Ms Samina Khan (PA to Director-Publishing), Mr KK Raman (Production Manager), Mr Rajesh Sharma (Production Coordinator), Ms Seema Dogra (Cover Designer), Mr Sumit (Graphic Designer), Mr Kapil Dev Sharma (DTP Operator) and Mr Sarvesh Kumar Singh (Proofreader) of M/s Jaypee Brothers' typesetting unit, New Delhi, India.

Our sincere thanks to Mr Venugopal V and Mr Vasudev H of M/s Jaypee Brothers' Bengaluru Branch, for taking this book to every corner of Karnataka.

Contents

CHAPTER 1

Thanatology

Thanatology, (from Greek thanatos, "death") the description or study of death and is concerned with the notion of death as the branch of science that deals with death in all its aspects.

The following changes are seen after death is classified as:

1. **Immediate Changes (Somatic death)**
2. **Early Changes (Cellular death)**
   a. **Skin changes**
      The blood circulation to the skin is stopped resulting in pallor and loss of elasticity.

   b. **Eye changes**
      An early change in eye seen as opacity of cornea and flaccidity of eyeball due to loss of intra-ocular tension, which progressively comes down to zero in about 2 hours.

   c. **Algor mortis (Postmortem cooling)**
      Is a progressive loss of heat due to; conduction, convection and radiation after death resulting in cooling of body.

   d. **Livor mortis (Postmortem lividity)**
      A passive pooling imparts reddish-purple or bluish discoloration of skin in dependent parts of the dead body is called as livor mortis with "contact flattening" on pressure areas of the body.

   e. **Rigor mortis (Postmortem rigidity)**
      A state of stiffening of muscles after death due to physiochemical process due to ATP is progressively and irreversibly destroyed by dephosphorylating and deamination leading to accumulation of lactates and phosphates in the muscles.

Conditions simulating Rigor Mortis
Heat stiffening: Temperature $> 65°C$
Cold stiffening: Temperature $< 3.5°C$
Gas stiffening: After putrefaction sets in.

Cadaveric Spasm/Instantaneous Rigor
In cases of sudden death from excitement, fear, severe pain, exhaustion etc. muscles that were contracted during life become stiff and rigid immediately after death without passing through stage of primary flaccidity due to which exact attitude of person at the time of death is preserved usually limited to single group of muscles frequently involving hands as seen here. This condition is known as Cadaveric Spasm or Instantaneous Rigor or Cataleptic Rigidity of the body.

3. Late Changes (Decomposition)

a. **Putrefaction:** Early sign of decomposition is greenish discoloration on right iliac fossa due to hemolysis of red blood cells and the liberated hemoglobin is converted into sulfmethemoglobin by hydrogen sulfide gas may be seen around 12–18 hours after death.

b. **Saponification (Adipocere)** ⎫
c. **Mummification** ⎬ Modified form of Putrefaction
                       ⎭

Skeletonization is the removal of tissues from the bones or skeleton, it may be *complete*; where all soft tissues are removed and *partial*, where only a few portions of the bones are exposed.

Artefacts

It may be regarded as any change caused or feature introduced in the natural state of the body that is likely to be misinterpreted at autopsy. These injuries may be produced by aquatic bites, ants and scavengers, etc.

Postmortem artefacts are due to any changes caused or features introduced in a body after death.

It is duty of medicolegal expert to differentiate artefacts from that of injuries thereby preventing false interpretation of finding and misleading of investigation.

Types of Artefacts

A. Resuscitation artefacts
B. Agonal artefacts
C. Postmortem artefacts due to:
   a. Improper handling of the body
   b. Postmortem changes
   c. Refrigeration in cold chamber
   d. Decomposition
   e. Animal and insect bites
   f. Autopsy surgeon induced
   g. Embalming
   h. Exhumation.

Forensic Entomology (Entomology of Cadaver)

Entomology: Study of insects.
Forensic entomology: Use of insect knowledge in the investigation of crime, used in estimation of time since death or postmortem interval (PMI).
Principle: As the insects arrive on the body soon after death, estimating age of insects can help in estimation of postmortem interval (PMI).
Based on: 1. Directly from the life cycle
             2. Waves of succession! Time of arrival of different species.
Stages of life cycle
Egg→Larvae→Pupa→Adult

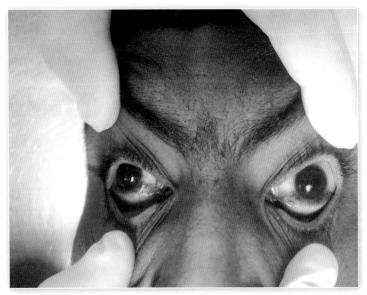

Figure 1   Tache Noire; an early postmortem change seen in eyes

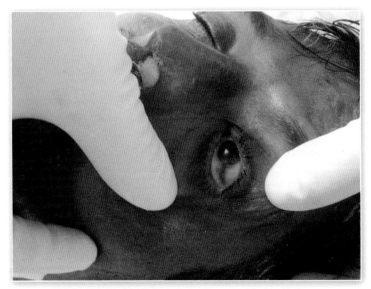

Figure 2   Tache Noire seen in the outer angle of left eye

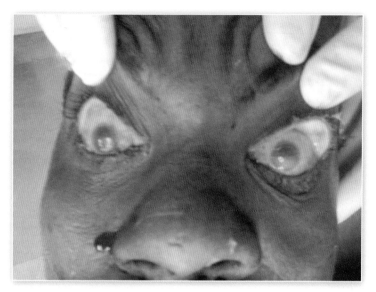

Figure 3   Clouding and haziness of cornea seen in both eyes

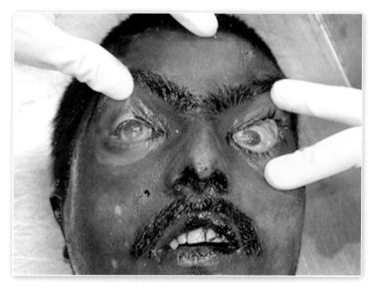

Figure 4   Sunken eyeballs and corneal opacity in both eyes

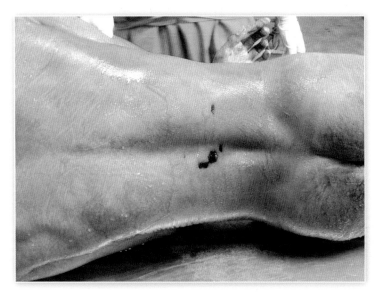

Figure 5   Postmortem lividity on the back

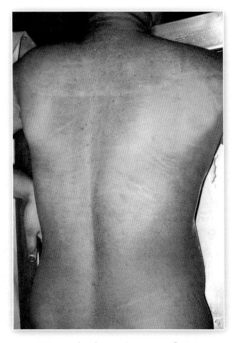

Figure 6   Postmortem lividity with contact flattening on the back

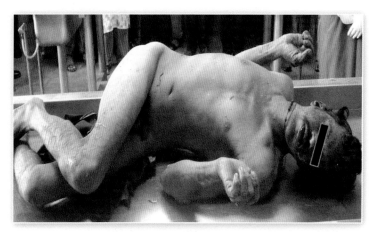

Figure 7   Entire body in rigor indicating the posture of the body after death

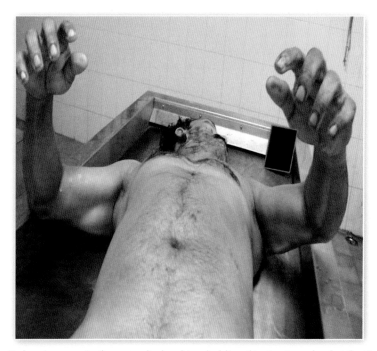

Figure 8   Cadaveric spasm in the upper limbs; driver holding the steering wheel at the time of death

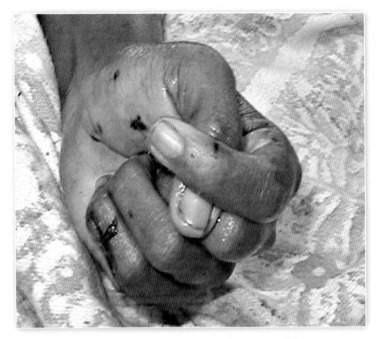

Figure 9 Instantaneous rigor of hand in a case of drowning

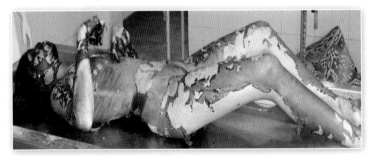

Figure 10 Heat stiffening of the body

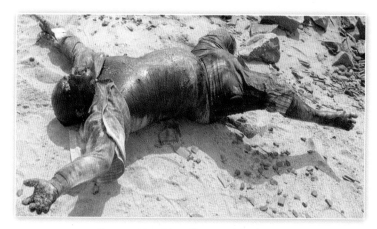

Figure 11   Gas stiffening of the body

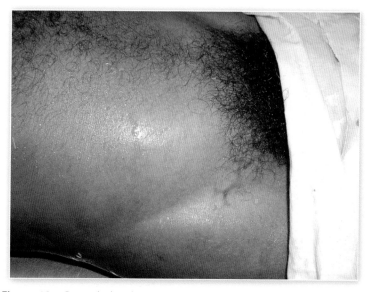

Figure 12   Greenish discoloration on the right iliac fossa and inguinal region

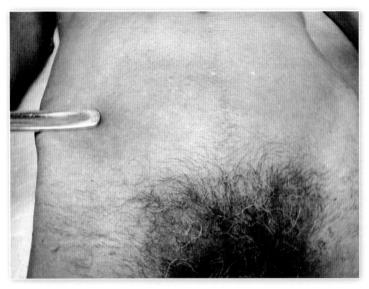

Figure 13 Greenish dicoloration of abdominal flanks

Marbling of skin in various parts of the body, due to invasion of microorganisms and formation of sulfmethemoglobin and thereby staining the blood vessels and then being prominent giving a marbled appearance to the skin may be seen around 24–36 hours after death **(Figs 14 to 19)**.

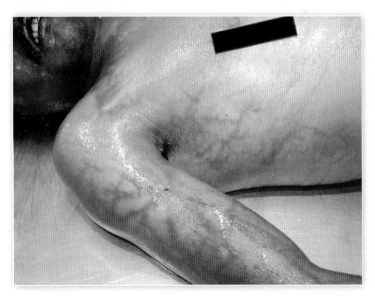

Figure 14 Marbling seen in right upper arm and right chest wall

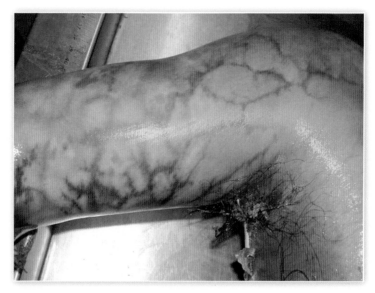

Figure 15   Marbling seen in axilla and right shoulder

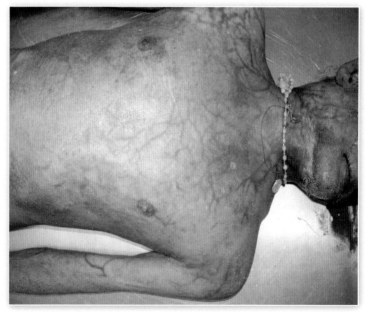

Figure 16   Marbling seen on upper part of the body

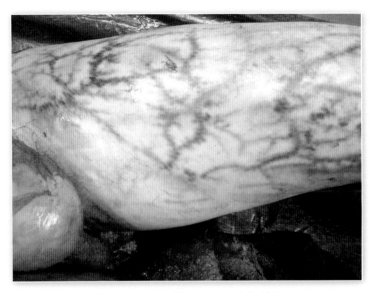

Figure 17   Marbling seen on left thigh

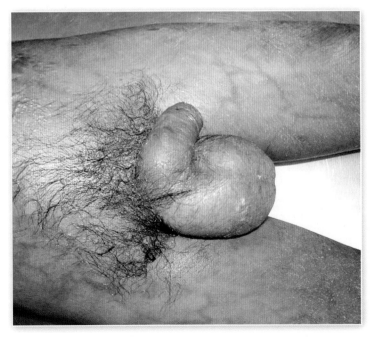

Figure 18   Marbling seen in left upper thigh and groin region

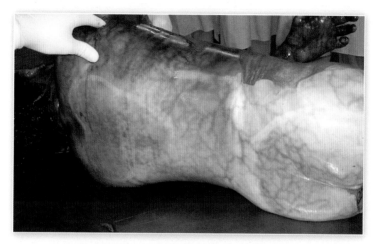

Figure 19 Marbling seen on the entire back

Autolysis of cells due to hydrolytic enzymes after death is observed as collection of fluids in between dermis and epidermis called ***postmortem blisters***. Loosening of epidermis from the underlying dermis is called ***skin slippage*** **(Figs 20 to 26)**.

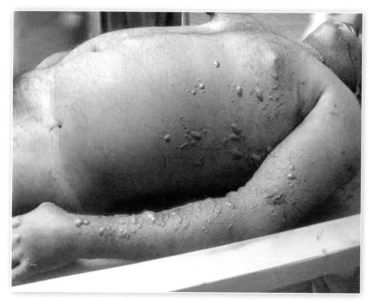

Figure 20 Postmortem blisters seen on left hand and left chest wall

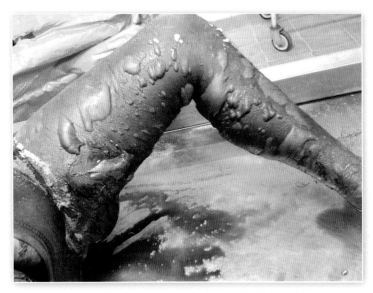

Figure 21   Postmortem blisters on left thigh and leg

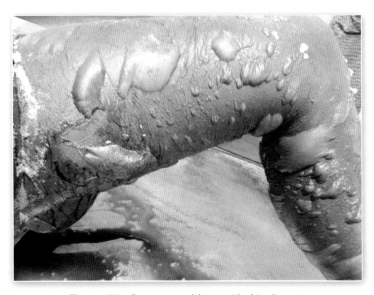

Figure 22   Postmortem blister with skin slippage

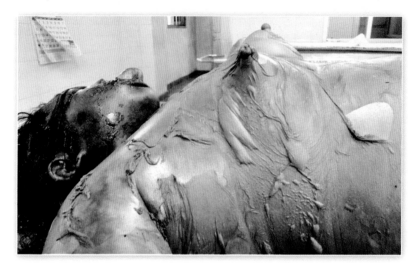

Figure 23   Postmortem blisters, skin slippage and erect nipples (gas stiffening)

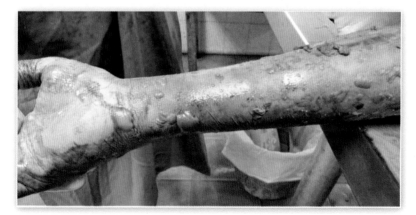

Figure 24   Postmortem blisters and skin slippage seen on the forearm and hand

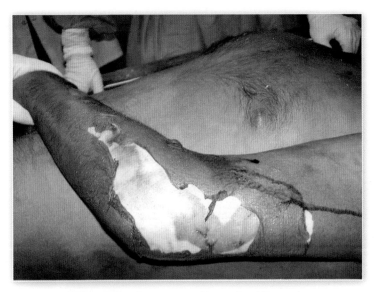

Figure 25 Postmortem skin peeling (slippage)

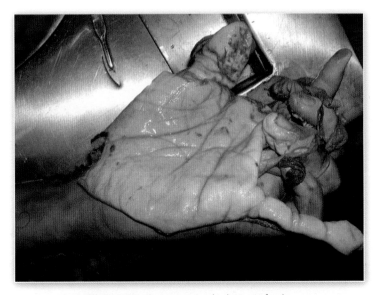

Figure 26 Postmortem degloving of palm

The putrefactive changes are seen with the advancement of postmortem interval such as; *color changes, bloating of face, protrusion of eye and tongue, distention of abdomen, and postmortem purging.* In males, *scrotal swelling* may be observed. During late decomposition process, foul smelling gases are liberated which are collected in the intestine in around 12–18 hours after death **(Figs 27 to 37)**.

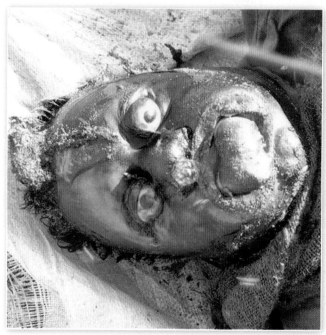

Figure 27   Bloated face with protruded eyeballs and tongue

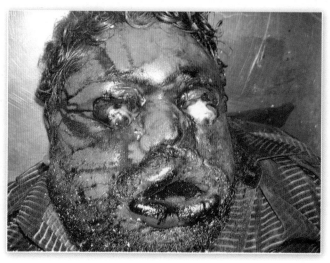

Figure 28   Bloated face, liquefaction of eyeballs and postmortem purge

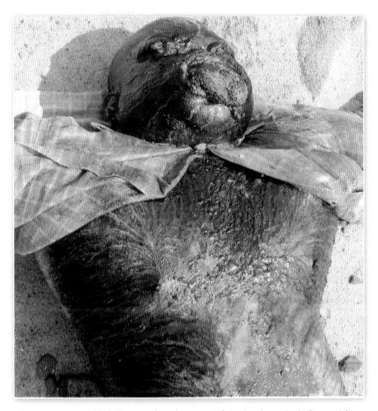

Figure 29   Reddish brown discoloration of the body with disfigured face

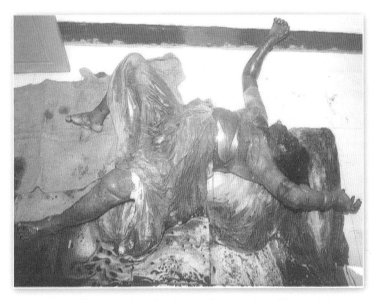

Figure 30   Gas stiffening and reddish brown discoloration of the body (crime scene)

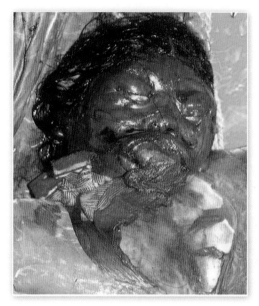

Figure 31   Disfigured face with protrusion of the tongue

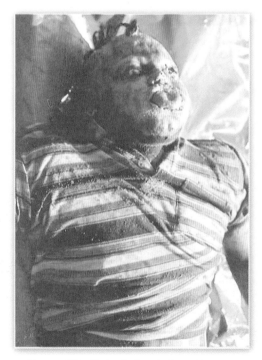

Figure 32   Protruded eyeballs and tongue

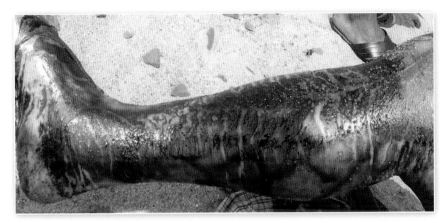

Figure 33   Reddish brown color changes

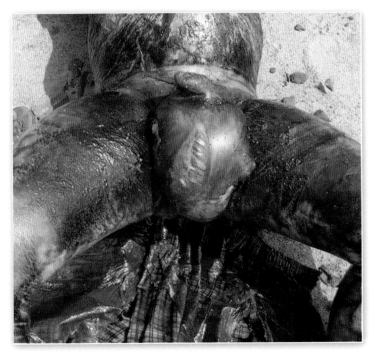

Figure 34   Distended scrotum with reddish brown color changes of the body

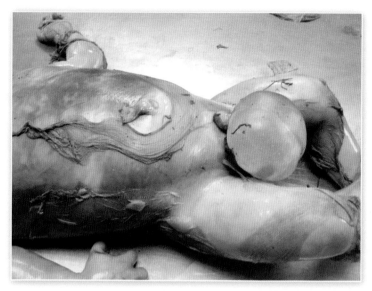

Figure 35   Decomposition showing scrotal swelling and skin slippage over abdomen in infant

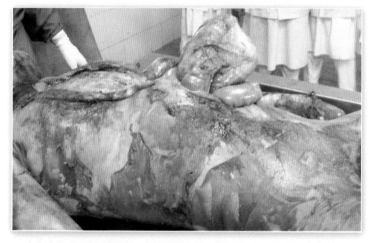

Figure 36   Protrusion of intestines on opening the abdominal cavity

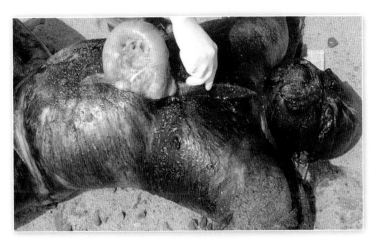

Figure 37 Protrusion of intestines on opening the abdominal cavity (autopsy conducted at the crime scene)

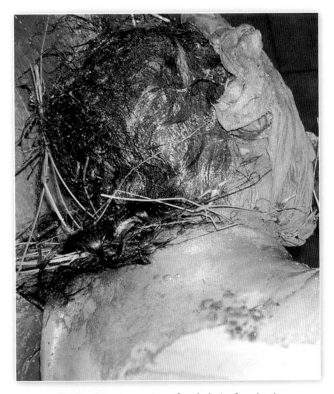

Figure 38 Loosening of scalp hair after death

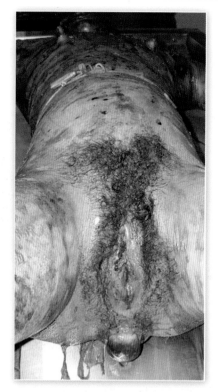

Figure 39   Postmortem prolapse of rectum

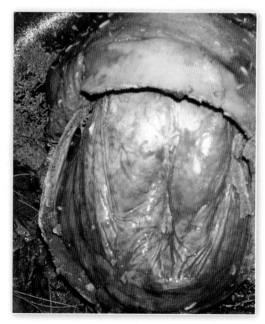

Figure 40   Intact, discolored and collapsed dura suggestive of underlying liquefied brain

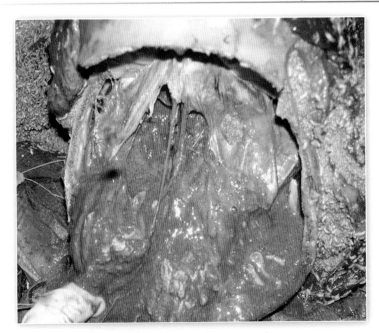

Figure 41 Liquefied discolored brain on removal of the dura

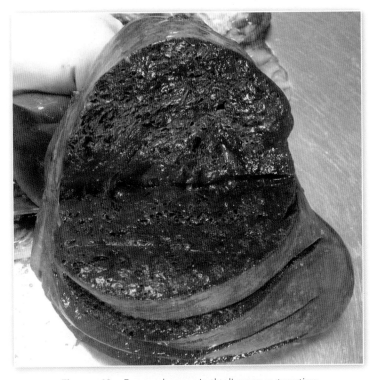

Figure 42 Foamy changes in the liver on cut section

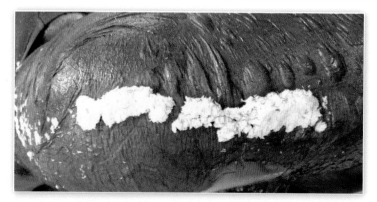

Figure 43   White clusters of eggs on the skin

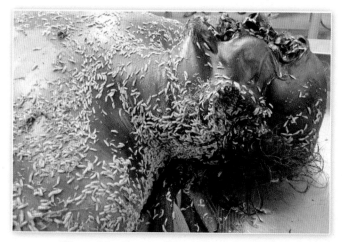

Figure 44   Clusters of maggots over the body

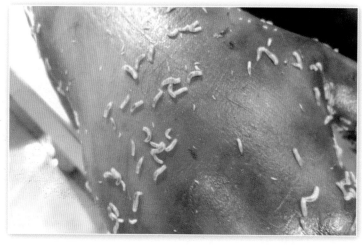

Figure 45   Maggots of varying sizes on the body

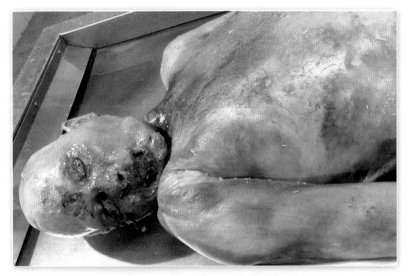

Figure 46 Adipocere formation of the body

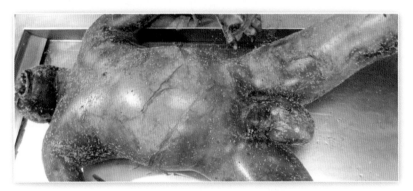

Figure 47 Adipocere with maggots

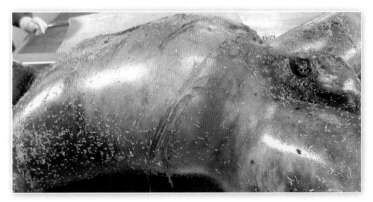

Figure 48 Adipocere over the abdomen and thigh with maggots

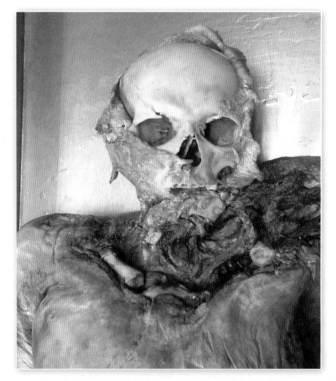

Figure 49 Partial skeletonization of the body

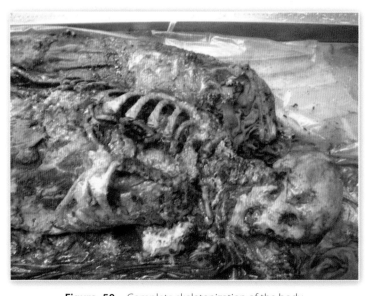

Figure 50 Complete skeletonization of the body

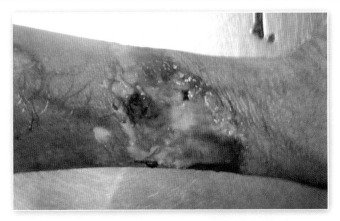

Figure 51 Artefact caused by aquatic animal

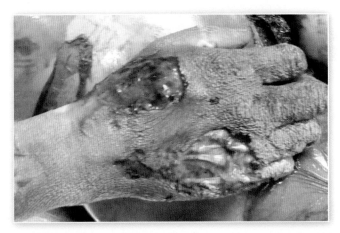

Figure 52 Artefacts on the back of hand caused by aquatic animal bites

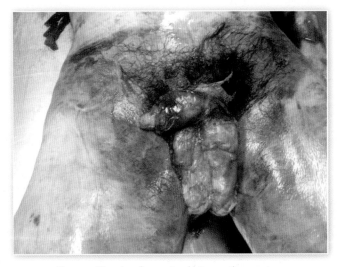

Figure 53 Artefact animal bite on the scrotum

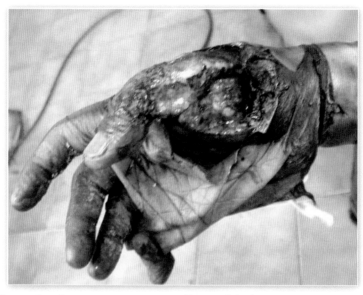

Figure 54   Postmortem aquatic animal bite and degloving seen in right hand

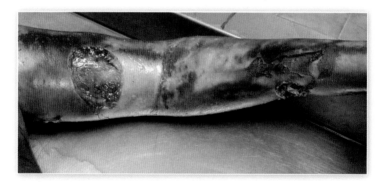

Figure 55   Postmortem rodent bite with nibbled margins

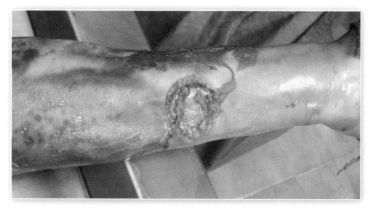

Figure 56   Artefact with nibbled margins caused by rodent bite

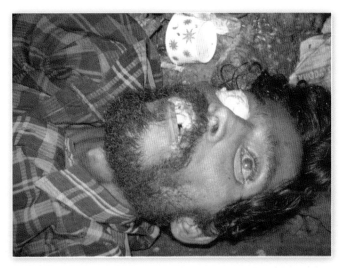

Figure 57   Enucleation of right eyeball due to rodent bite with nibbled margins

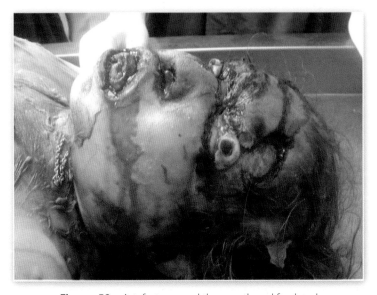

Figure 58   Artefacts around the mouth and forehead

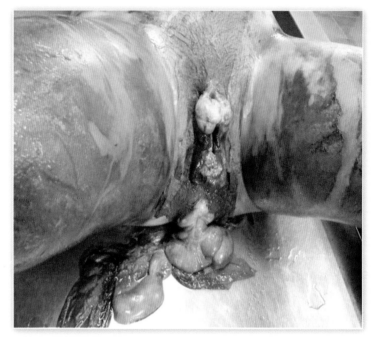

Figure 59 Artefact of female external genitalia (animal bite)

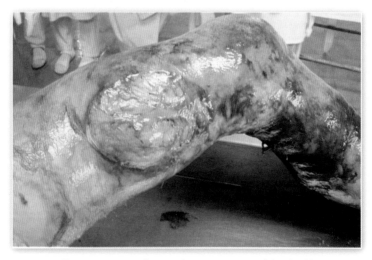

Figure 60 Artefact on the inner aspect of the thigh

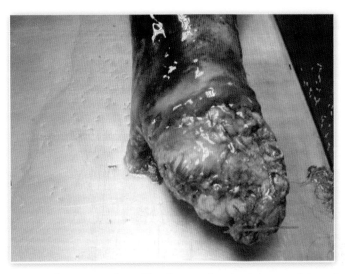

Figure 61   Postmortem loss of foot by aquatic animals (a case of drowning)

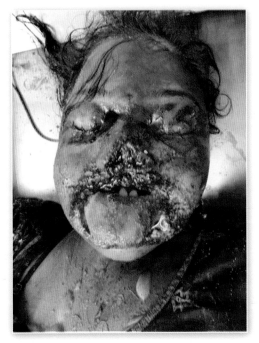

Figure 62   Postmortem animal bites around the mouth and nostrils

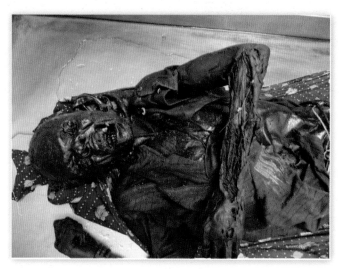

Figure 63   Mummified body

CHAPTER 2

Mechanical Injuries

Trauma, injury, hurt and wound may appear similar but they differ in medical and legal context. Section 44 of Indian Penal Code (IPC) defines injury as "any harm whatever illegally caused to a person in body, mind, reputation and property". Section 319 of IPC defines hurt as "whoever causes bodily pain, disease or infirmity to any other person, is said to cause hurt". As per WHO, trauma is an insult to the state of wellbeing, which can be physical or mental. Medicolegally wound can be defined as any lesion external or internal caused by violence with or without loss of continuity of skin.

Mechanical injuries can be defined as "Damage to any part of the body due to application of mechanical force".

CLASSIFICATION OF MECHANICAL INJURIES

Mechanical injuries can be classified based on the nature of force applied as:
1. **Injuries due to blunt force trauma**
   A. **Abrasions**: Loss of superficial layers of skin or mucous membrane. They can be classified based on manner of causation as:
      a. Pressure abrasion
      b. Graze abrasion
      c. Imprint/impact/patterned abrasion
      d. Scratch/Linear abrasion.
   B. **Contusions/bruises**: Extravascular collection of blood due to damage of blood vessels without loss of continuity of skin.
   C. **Lacerations**: Rupture or tear of skin or deeper tissues. They can be classified based on manner of causation as:
      a. Split/Incised looking laceration
      b. Stretch laceration
      c. Avulsed/grind laceration
      d. Tear laceration
      e. Cut laceration.
   D. **Fractures**: Breakage of bone due to direct or indirect forces. They can be classified as:
      a. Linear fracture
      b. Comminuted fracture
      c. Penetrating fracture.

2. **Injuries due to sharp force trauma**
   A. **Incised wound/cut/slash/slice:** Clean cut separation of skin and/or deeper tissues caused by sharp cutting weapon without contusion and crushing of margins. Here length is the largest dimension.
   B. **Chop wound:** Clean cut separation of skin and/or deeper tissues caused by sharp cutting weapon without contusion and crushing of margins. It is usually caused by heavy sharp cutting weapons.
   C. **Stab wound/puncture:** Piercing wounds caused by sharp pointed objects. Margins may be clean cut or contused depending on weapon. They appear like incised wound but here depth is the largest dimension. They can be classified as:
      a. Penetrating wound: Only entry wound present but no exit.
      b. Perforating wound: Both entry and exit wounds present.

Pressure abrasions over elbow, knees, leg, thigh and back. These abrasions are seen commonly in cases of road traffic accident and fall signifying the site of impact **(Figs 1 to 5)**.

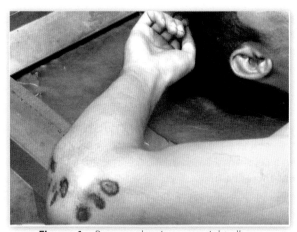

Figure 1 Pressure abrasions over right elbow

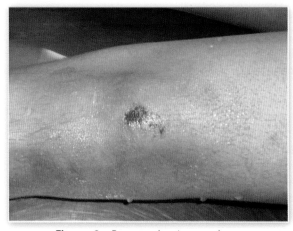

Figure 2 Pressure abrasion over knee

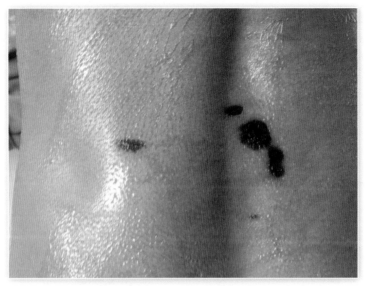

Figure 3   Reddish brown pressure abrasions over the back

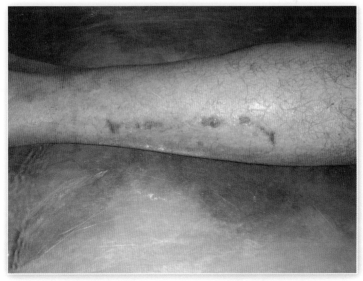

Figure 4   Reddish pressure abrasions over the leg

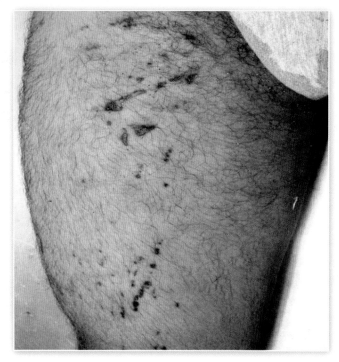

Figure 5 Multiple pressure abrasions on thigh

Abrasions in different stages of healing over leg, knee and elbow. Abrasions heal with scab formation, different color changes and stages of scab formation can tell about the time since injury **(Figs 6 to 9)**.

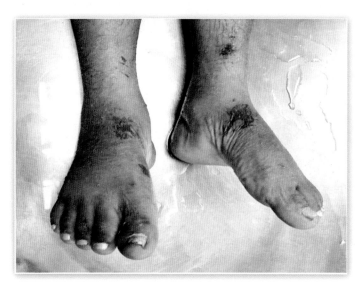

Figure 6 Abrasions with reddish brown scab over leg and foot

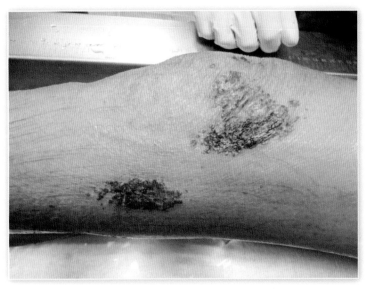

Figure 7   Partially healed abrasions with reddish brown scab

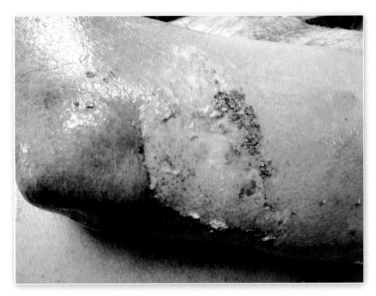

Figure 8   Partially healed abrasions with scab fallen off

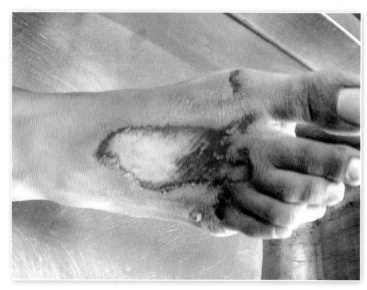

Figure 9 Partially healed abrasion

After death, abrasions are caused if the body is subjected to friction, or attacked by creatures like ants, aquatic animals, etc. They need to be differentiated from antemortem injuries by the absence of color changes and vital reaction **(Figs 10 to 13)**.

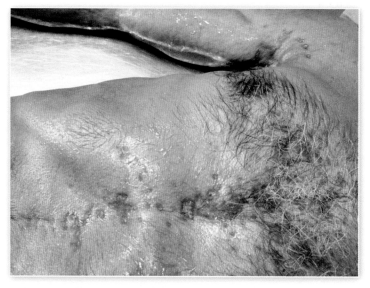

Figure 10 Ant bite marks on the front of trunk

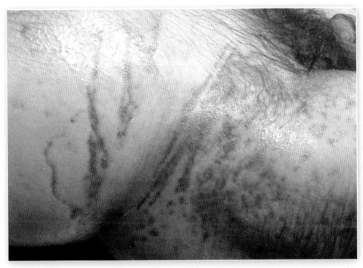

Figure 11 Ant bite marks

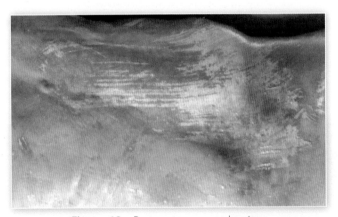

Figure 12 Postmortem graze abrasions

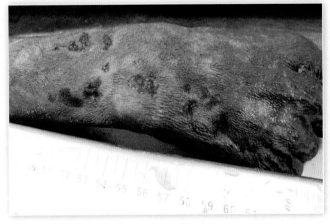

Figure 13 Postmortem abrasions on the wrist

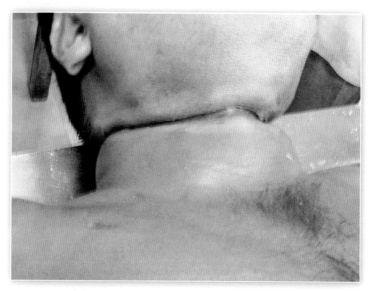

Figure 14 Pressure abrasion on the neck caused due to sustained pressure by ligature material

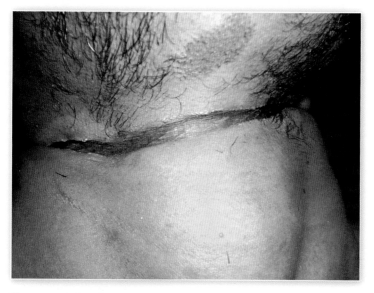

Figure 15 Deeply grooved imprint abrasion (ligature mark) on the neck

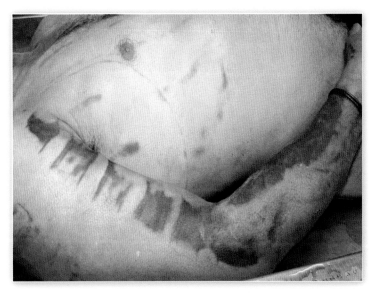

Figure 16 Tyre tread imprint abrasion over right upper limb

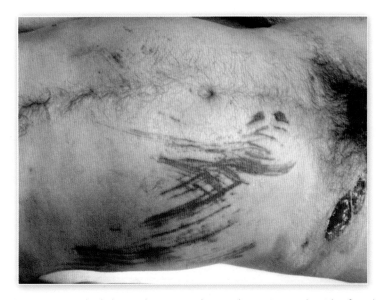

Figure 17 Multiple linear abrasions with a tear laceration on the side of trunk

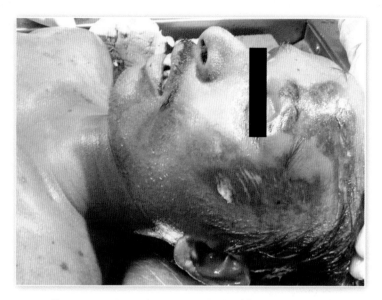

Figure 18   Graze abrasions over side of face and forehead

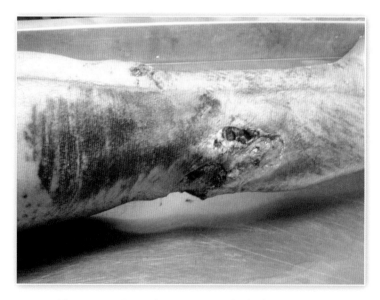

Figure 19   Graze abrasions over right thigh along with
laceration over upper part of leg

Graze abrasions are usually seen in cases of road traffic accidents when body slides over the rough surface. Grazes help to comment on the direction of impact. They are more prominent near origin of impact and gradually fades out towards the end. Brush burns are extreme forms of grazes, formed due to generation of heat resulting from severe friction between the body and rough surface **(Figs 20 to 26)**.

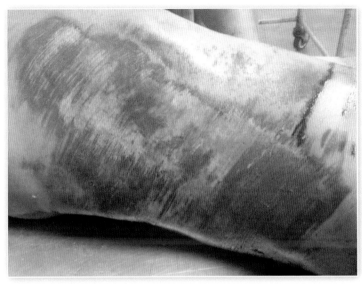

Figure 20   Graze abrasions over back

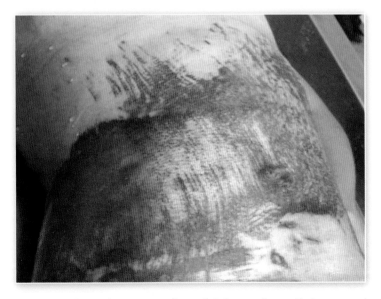

Figure 21   Graze abrasions over front of abdomen directed below upwards

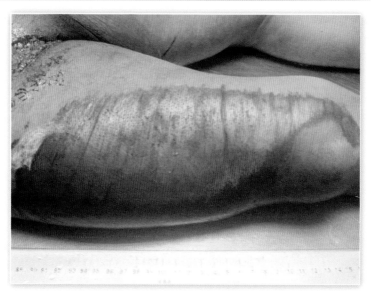

Figure 22   Brush burns on outer aspect of thigh

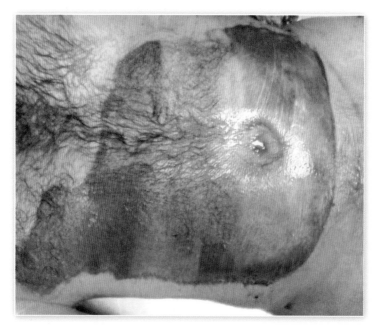

Figure 23   Brush Burns on abdomen

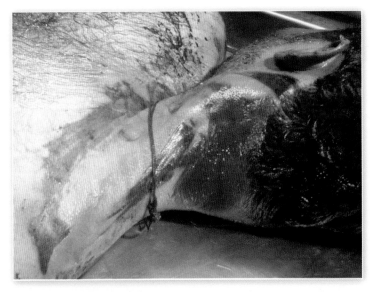

Figure 24   Brush burns over back of neck

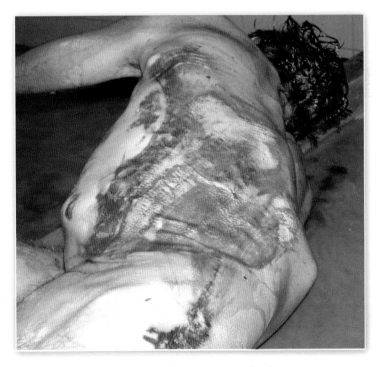

Figure 25   Brush burns over back

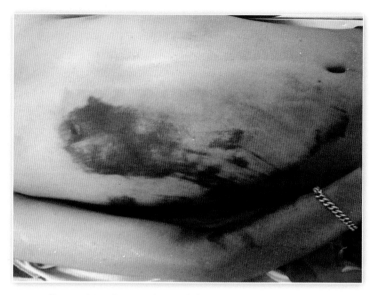

Figure 26　Contused grazed abrasion on the side of trunk

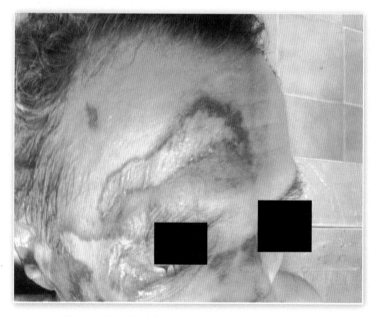

Figure 27　Partially healed abrasions over forehead

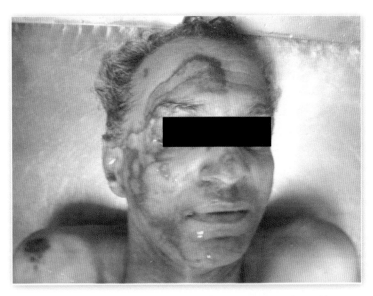

Figure 28 Abrasions over forehead, cheek, nose and shoulder

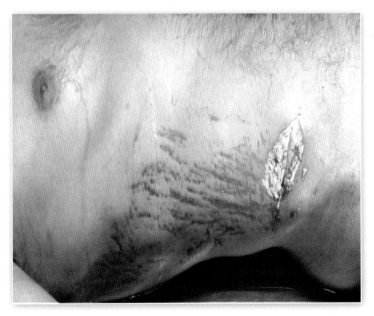

Figure 29 Multiple abrasions with tear laceration of the trunk

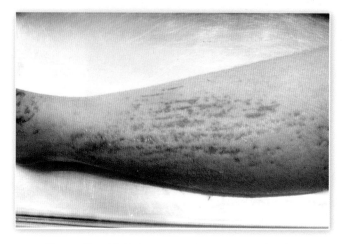

Figure 30   Multiple pressure abrasions over the shin

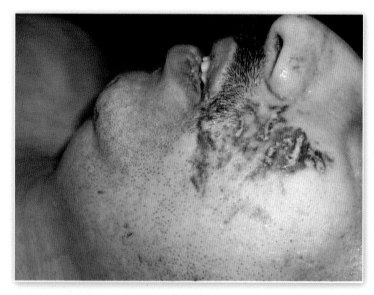

Figure 31   Abrasions with superficial lacerations over cheek

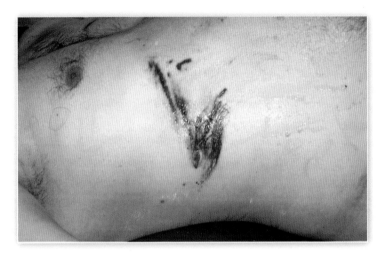

Figure 32   Contused abrasions on side of trunk

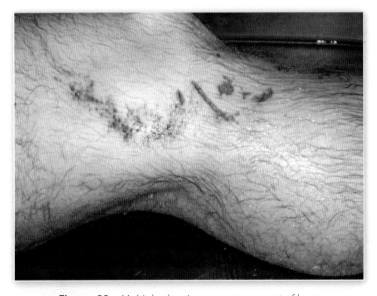

Figure 33   Multiple abrasions on outer aspect of knee

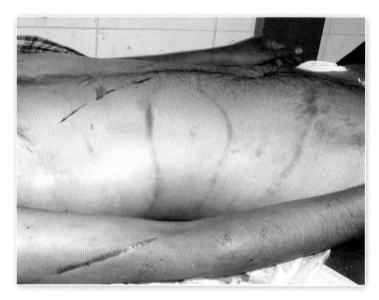

Figure 34   Multiple linear contusions over trunk

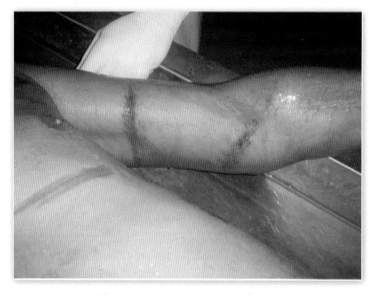

Figure 35   Contusions over left arm

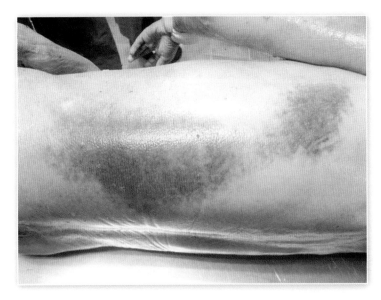

Figure 36   Contusion on the side of trunk

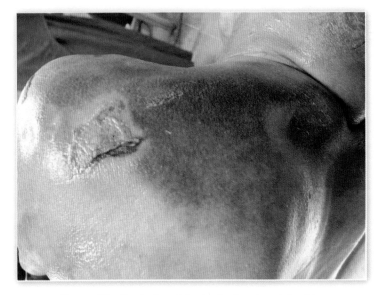

Figure 37   Contusion at the back of neck and shoulder

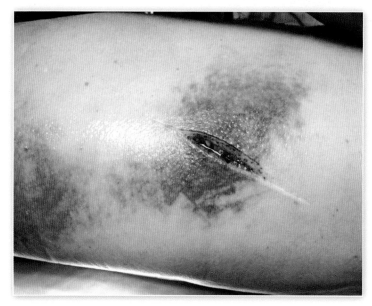

Figure 38   Contusion incised to show the extravasation of blood

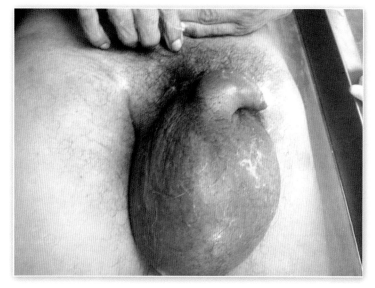

Figure 39   Scrotal hematoma

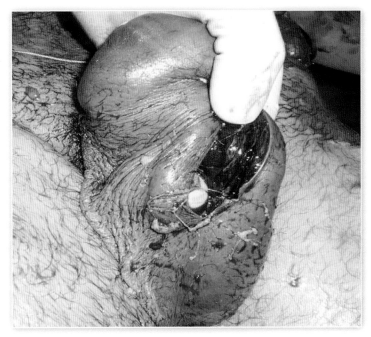

Figure 40   Scrotum dissected to show underlying hematoma

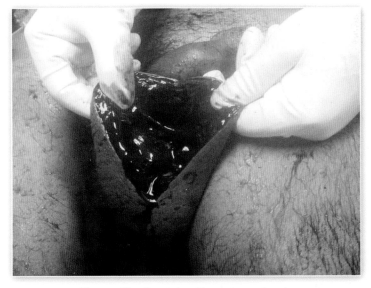

Figure 41   Contusion of scrotum and testis

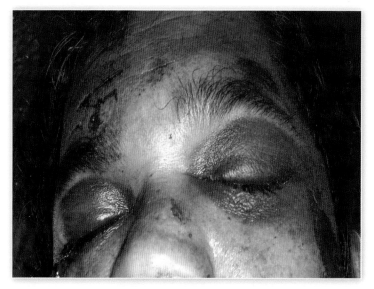

Figure 42   Bilateral black eyes (spectacle hematoma) caused due to extravasation of blood in periorbital space

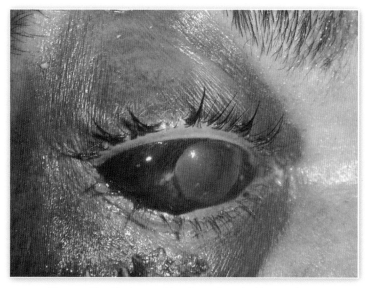

Figure 43   Black eye with sub-conjunctival hemorrhage

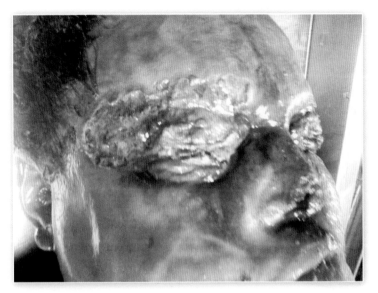

Figure 44 Postmortem lesions caused by aquatic animal bite

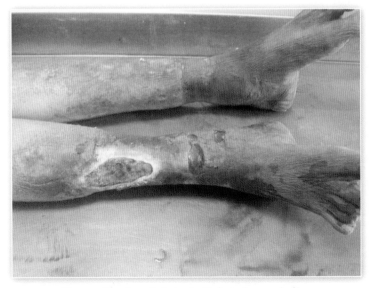

Figure 45 A partially healed infected wound of leg

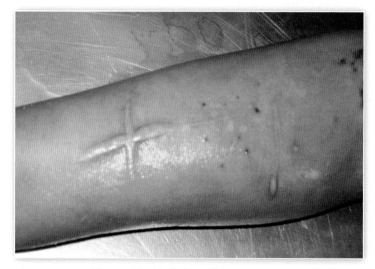

Figure 46   Healed scar (hesitation cuts)

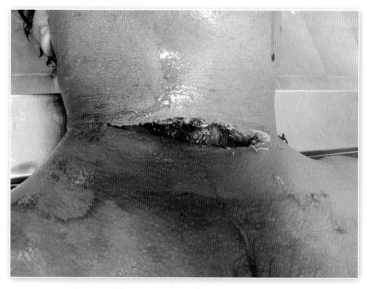

Figure 47   Cut throat injury

Defense cuts are inflicted when a person tries to ward off an attack, thus are commonly located on hands, forearms, etc. as these are the parts of body mostly used for defense. However, they can be seen on other parts as back, legs also depending upon the relative position of victim and assailant **(Figs 48 to 50)**.

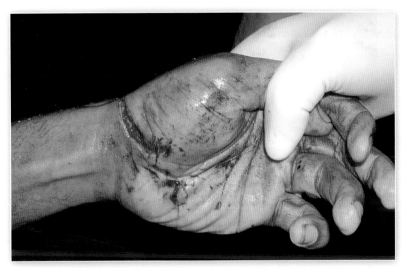

Figure 48   Incised wound (Defense cut) over left palm

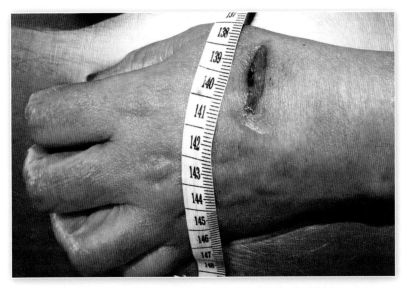

Figure 49   Incised wound (Defense cut) at the back of left hand

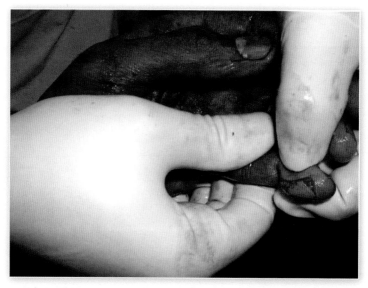

Figure 50   Incised wound (Defense cut) over finger

Incised wounds are caused by sharp weapons like knife, blade sword, etc. and have clear cut margins with clean cut underlying tissues, vessels and nerves **(Figs 51 to 56)**.

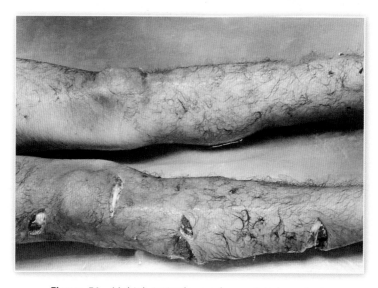

Figure 51   Multiple incised wounds over right lower limb

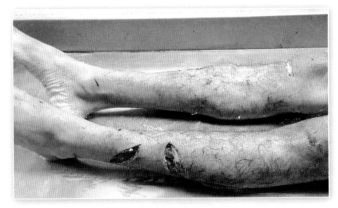

Figure 52 Incised wounds over left lower limb

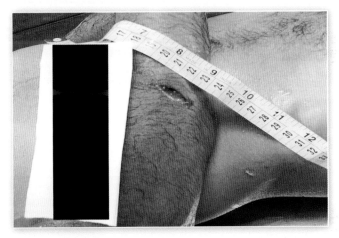

Figure 53 Incised wound over forearm

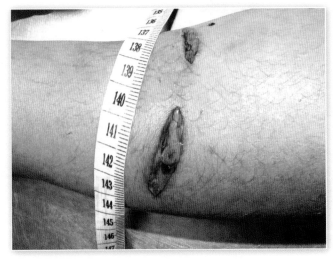

Figure 54 Incised wounds over leg

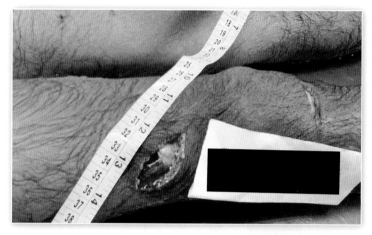

Figure 55   Incised wounds over right thigh and knee

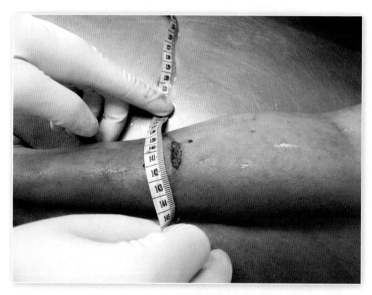

Figure 56   Incised wound over forearm

Chop wounds are caused by heavy sharp weapons like axe, sword, etc. Here margins are clean cut and contused with cutting and crushing of underlying muscles, bones, vessels and nerves **(Figs 57 to 64)**.

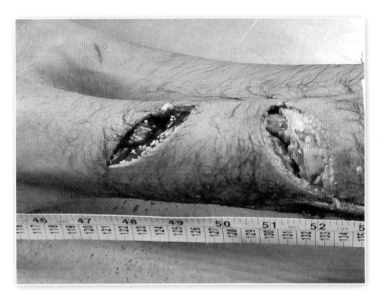

Figure 57 Chop wounds over shin

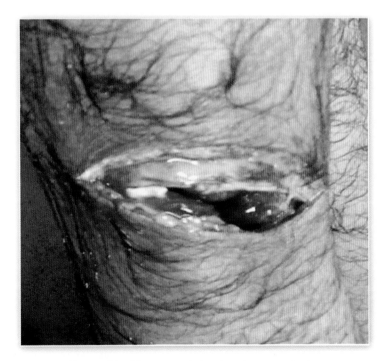

Figure 58 Chop wound showing clean cut margins

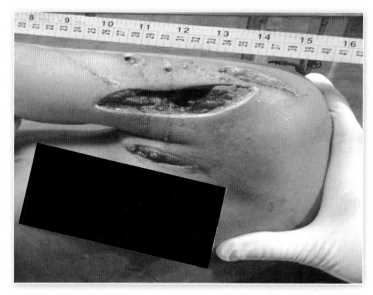

Figure 59   Chop wound at the back of left shoulder

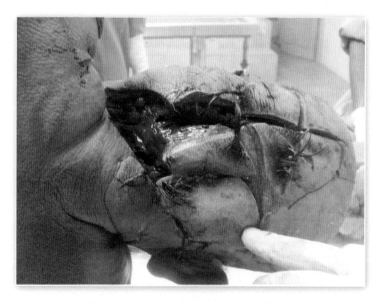

Figure 60   Multiple chop wounds of head

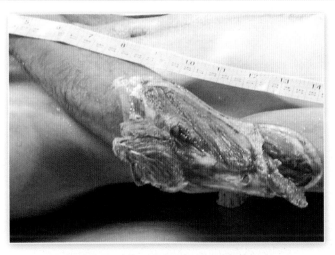

Figure 61   Chop wound of left upper limb

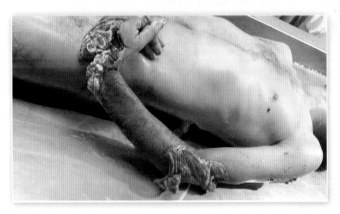

Figure 62   Chop wounds of left upper limb with partial amputation at wrist

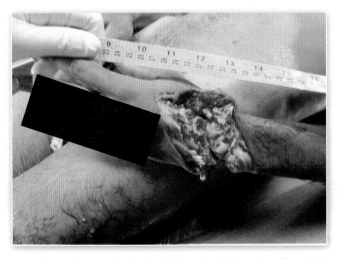

Figure 63   Chop wound at the back of left hand with beveling of underlying bone

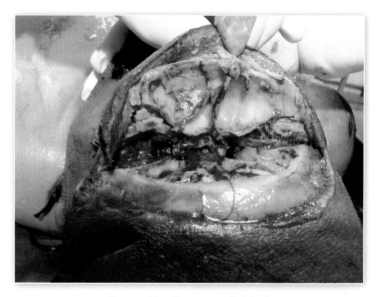

Figure 64 Chop wound of skull

Stab wounds are caused due to sharp or blunt penetrating weapon like knife, ice pick, sword, etc. Appearance is usually similar to incised wound but here depth is larger dimension as compared to length whereas in incised wounds length is more as compared to depth **(Figs 65 to 70)**.

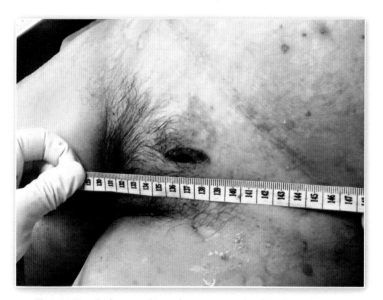

Figure 65 Stab wound in pubic region with adjoining contusion

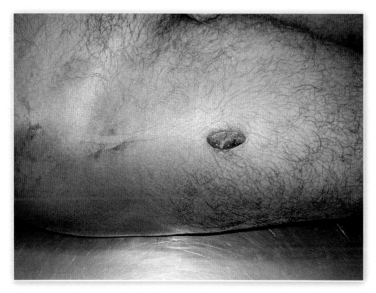

Figure 66   Stab wound over thigh

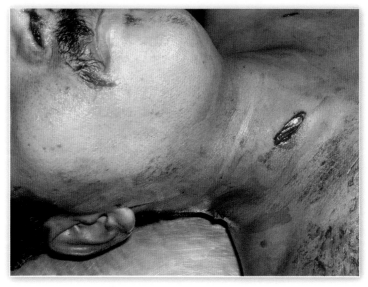

Figure 67   Stab wound over neck

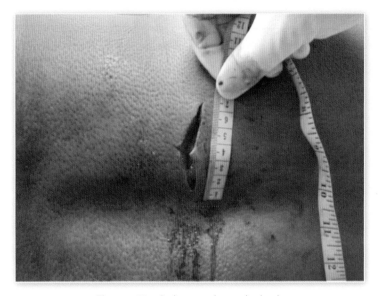

Figure 68 Stab wound over the back

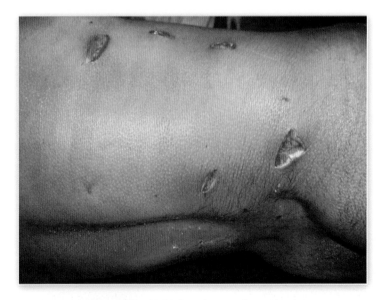

Figure 69 Multiple stab wounds over back

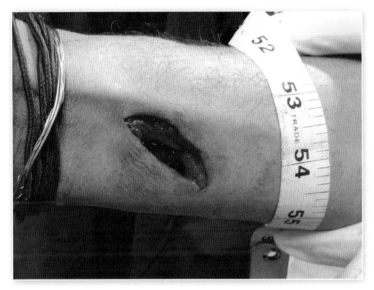

Figure 70   Stab wound of forearm with underlying tissue damage

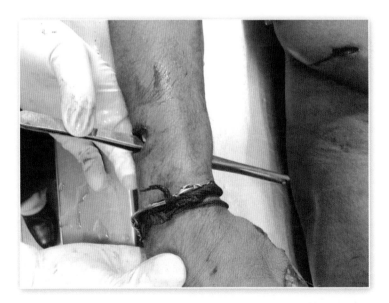

Figure 71   Demonstration of perforating stab wound of forearm

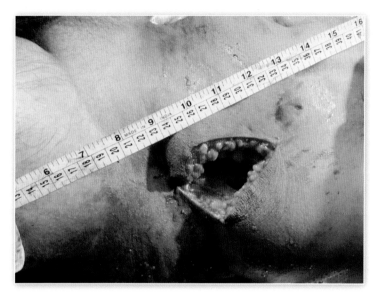

Figure 72   Stab wound with irregular margins

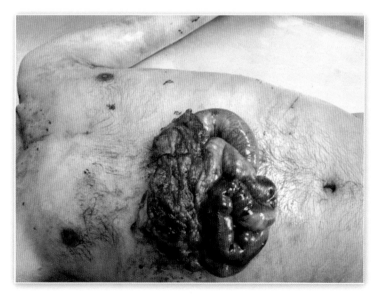

Figure 73   Stab wound of abdomen with protrusion of loops of intestine

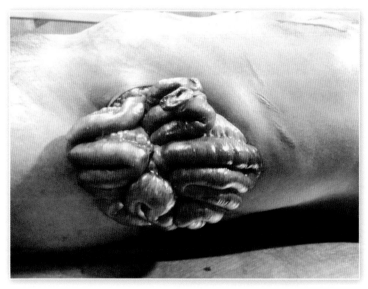

Figure 74   Stab wound of abdomen with evisceration

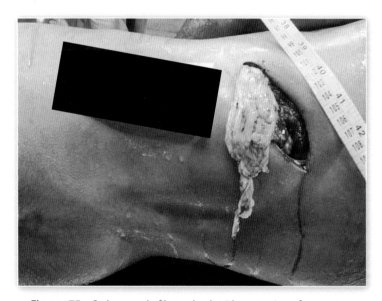

Figure 75   Stab wound of lower back with protrusion of mesentery

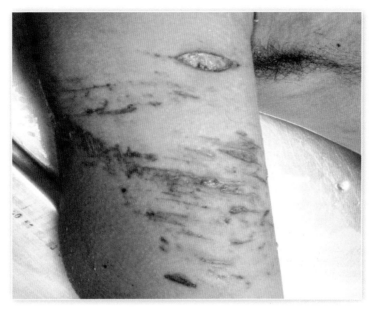

Figure 76   Incised wound with multiple superficial lacerations

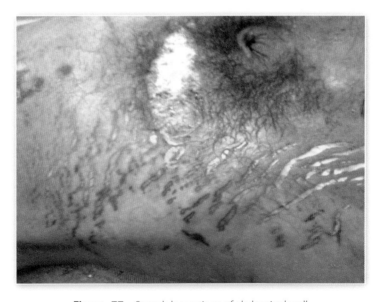

Figure 77   Stretch lacerations of abdominal wall

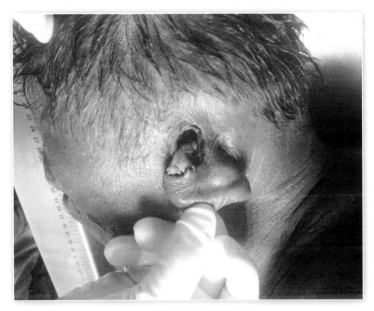

Figure 78 Avulsed laceration of pinna

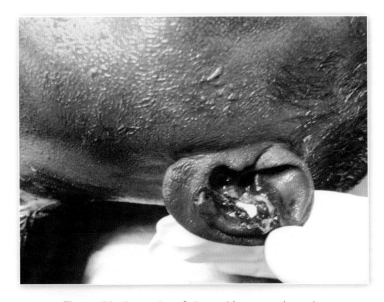

Figure 79 Laceration of pinna with contused margins

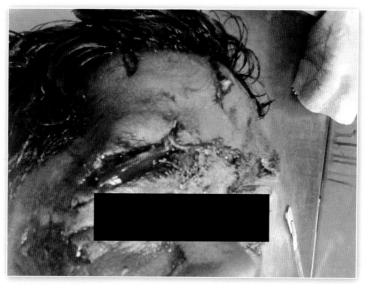

Figure 80   Multiple lacerations over forehead

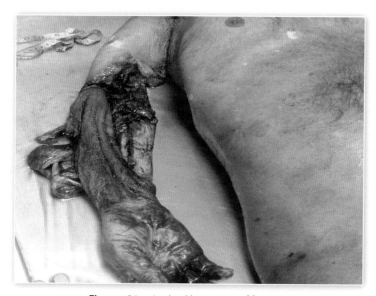

Figure 81   Avulsed laceration of forearm

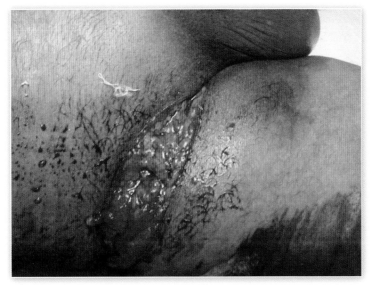

Figure 82   Stretch laceration of groin

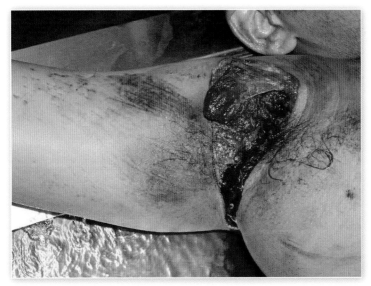

Figure 83   Laceration of right axilla and graze abrasion of right arm

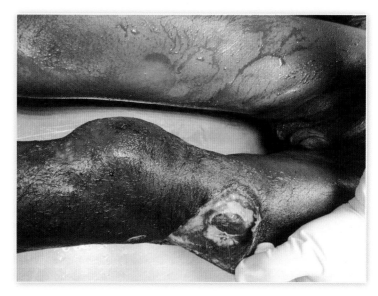

Figure 84   Avulsed laceration of left thigh

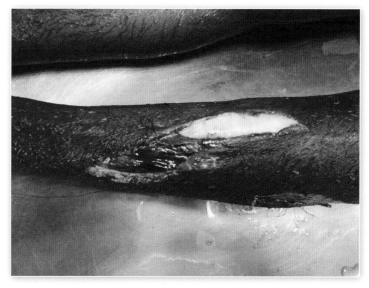

Figure 85   Incised looking laceration over shin

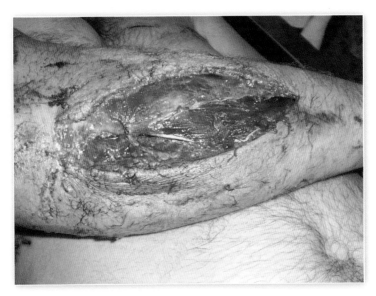

Figure 86 Laceration of forearm with bridging of tissue

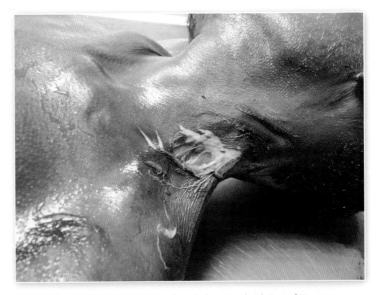

Figure 87 Laceration of neck showing bridging of tissues

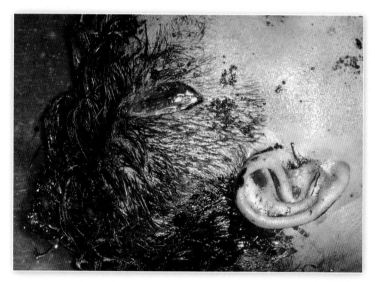

Figure 88   Split laceration on right side of head

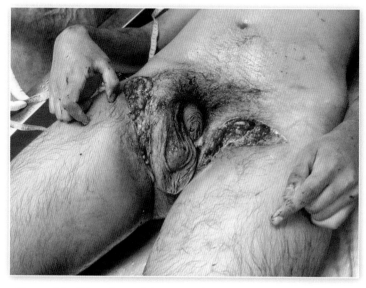

Figure 89   Bilateral stretch laceration due to run over by heavy vehicle

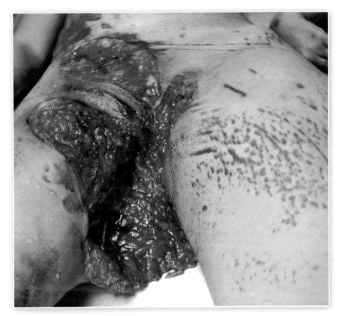

Figure 90   Avulsed laceration of right thigh and perineum along with stretch lacerations of left thigh

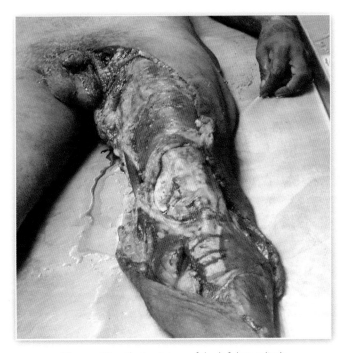

Figure 91   Flaying injury of the left lower limb

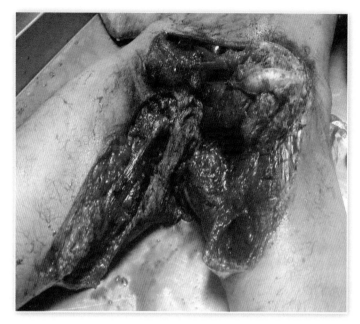

Figure 92 Avulsed laceration with degloving of male external genitalia

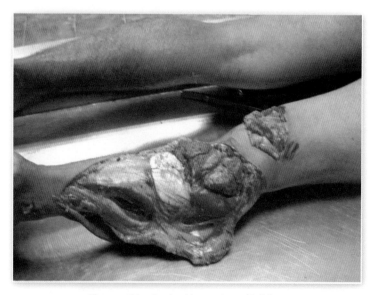

Figure 93 Avulsed laceration of left leg

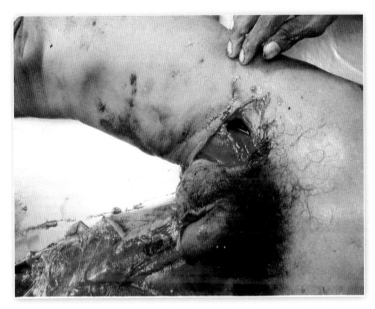

Figure 94 Laceration of right groin along with contusion of right thigh and avulsion of left thigh

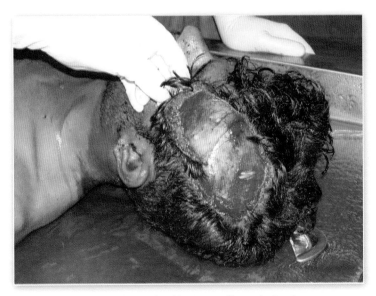

Figure 95 Avulsed laceration (flaying) of scalp.

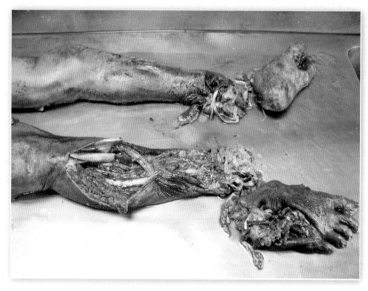

Figure 96   Complete transection and crush injury to lower limbs in railway accident

CHAPTER 3

Thermal Injuries

Thermal injuries are caused by exposure to excessive heat/cold. In tropical climate, generalized effects of high temperatures may be seen in form of heat cramps, heat prostration, or heat hyperpyrexia. Localized effects of heat may be observed in form of burns resulting from dry heat and scalds occurring as a result of moist heat. Similarly, extreme degree of cold can cause hypothermia or a frost bite, trench foot and immersion foot locally.

Injuries caused due to the localized effects of heat are classified based on the extent of damage to the skin and underlying tissues. A few of these classifications include Dupuytren's classification, Hebra's classification, Wilson's classification, and Modern classification. The effects and outcome of burns depend on various factors such as the degree of heat, duration of exposure, extent and parts of the body involved, and age and sex of the individual. Death in cases of fatal burns may be immediate, early or delayed. The immediate cause of death may be neurogenic shock, suffocation or secondary injuries while septicemia remains the most common cause of delayed death in thermal burns.

Burns produced by flame cause singeing of hairs, and blackening of skin. Blister formation and skin slippage are other associated features. Pus and slough formation is a delayed change that is often related with septicemia as the cause of death. The pressure areas are known to escape the effects of heat. Identification features such as tattoo marks are retained even when superficial layer is damaged in burns.

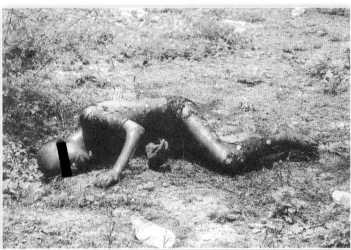

Figure 1 A charred body found in an open area

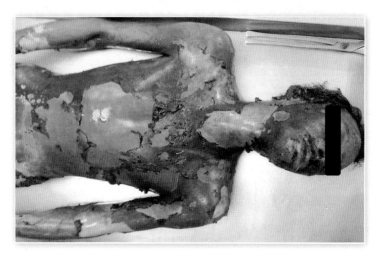

Figure 2 Burnt areas with evidence of blackening, peeling and reddening of skin

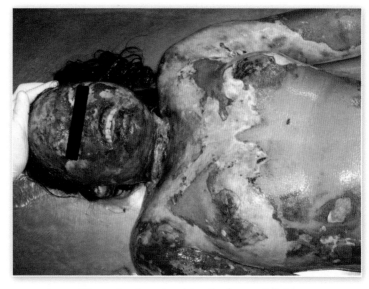

Figure 3 Burns involving the face and chest

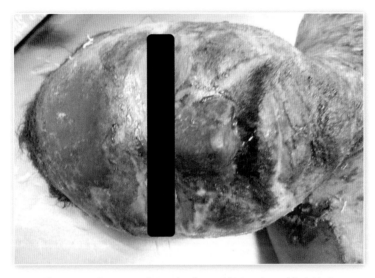

Figure 4 Burns involving the face with singeing of facial hair

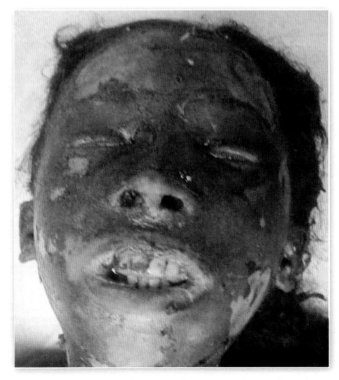

Figure 5 Blackening of face, singeing of scalp and facial hair with soot deposition over teeth

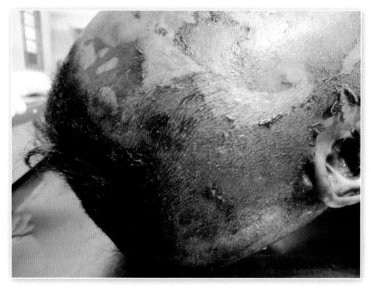

Figure 6   Singeing of scalp hair

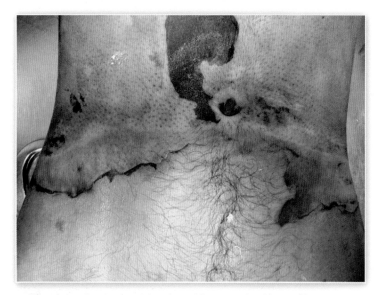

Figure 7   Demarcation (erythema) between healthy and burnt area

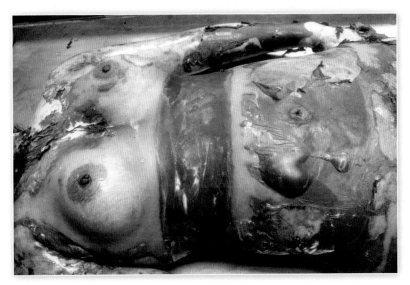

Figure 8 Blackening of skin with blister formation over trunk and spared areas over chest

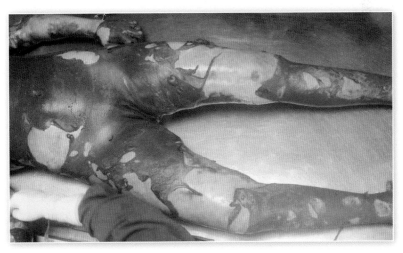

Figure 9 Blackening and peeling of skin in burns

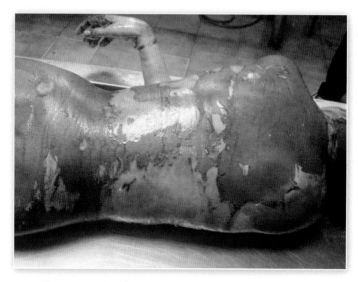

Figure 10   Reddening and peeling of the skin at the back

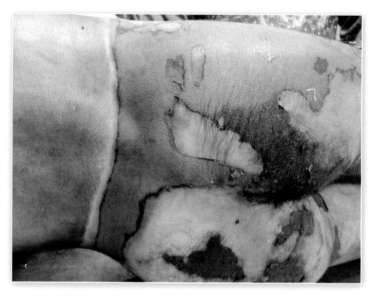

Figure 11   Burn areas with red line of demarcation

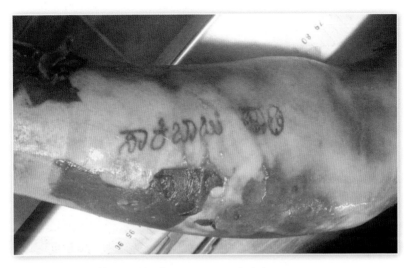

Figure 12 Intact tattoo marks in burn areas

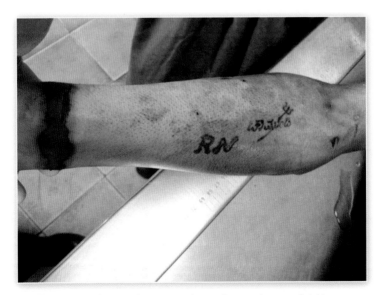

Figure 13 Retained tattoo mark over forearm in superficial burns

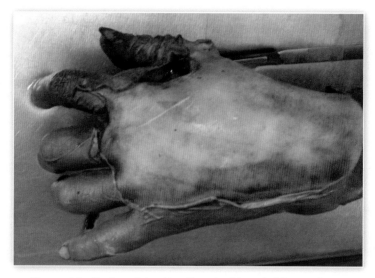

Figure 14 Peeling of the skin of hands with underlying erythema

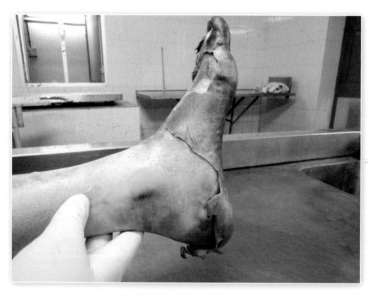

Figure 15 Peeling of the skin of sole in burns

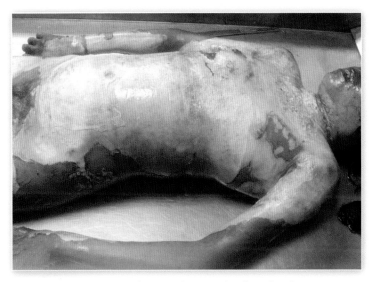

Figure 16 Deep burns with greenish yellow discoloration

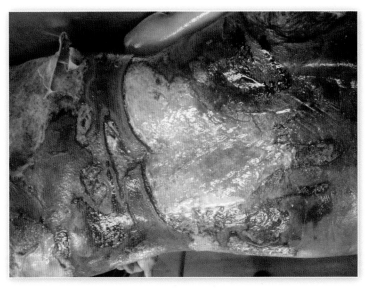

Figure 17 Infected areas over back in burns

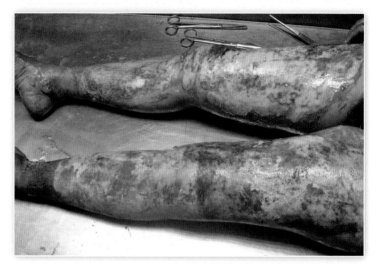

Figure 18   Pus and slough formation over infected areas in burns

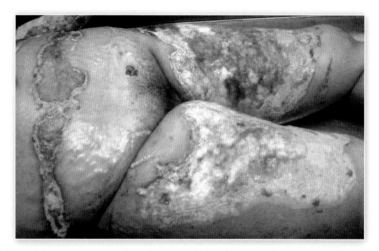

Figure 19   Burn areas showing pus and slough formation with partial healing

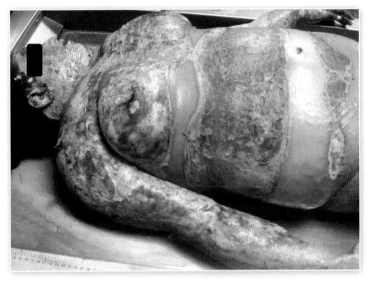

Figure 20 Burn areas with pus and slough formation

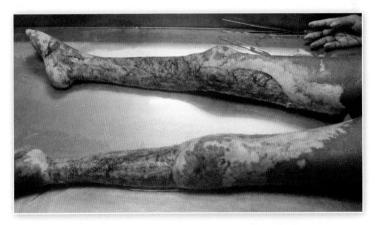

Figure 21 Infected burn areas over lower limbs

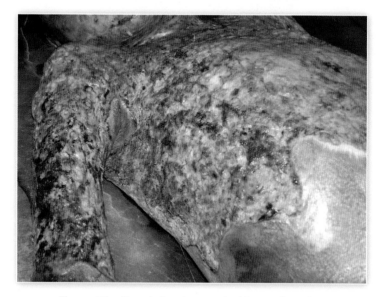

Figure 22   Granulation tissue and evidence of scarring

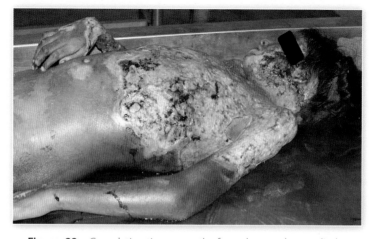

Figure 23   Granulation tissue over the face, chest and upper limbs

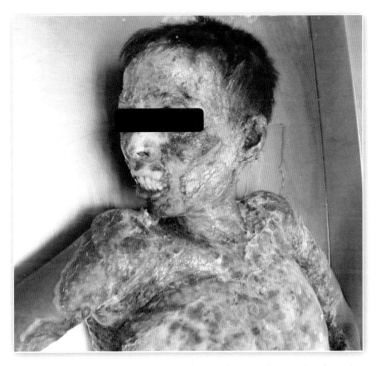

Figure 24 Granulation tissue over the face and upper chest with infected areas

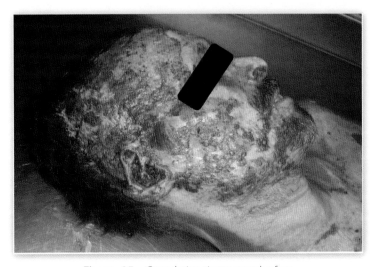

Figure 25 Granulation tissue over the face

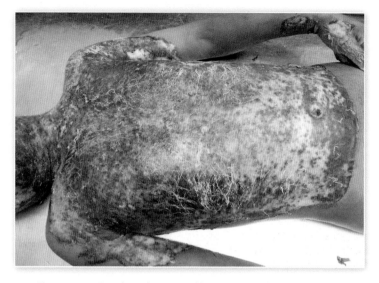

Figure 26 Dried parchmentized burn areas with partial healing

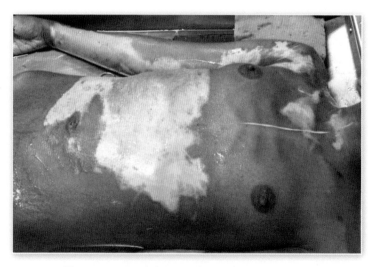

Figure 27 Healed areas in burns showing scarring

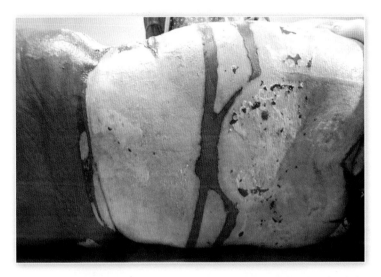

Figure 28   Spared areas in burns corresponding to the straps of underclothing

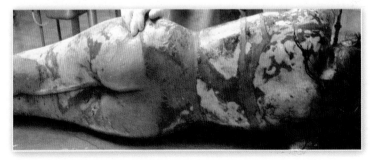

Figure 29   Spared areas in burns corresponding to the undergarments

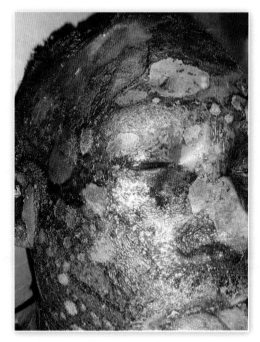

Figure 30   Singeing of scalp and facial hair in extensive burns involving face

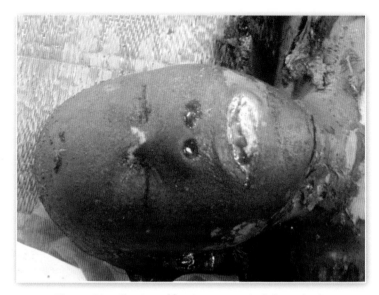

Figure 31   Charring of face in an extensively burnt body

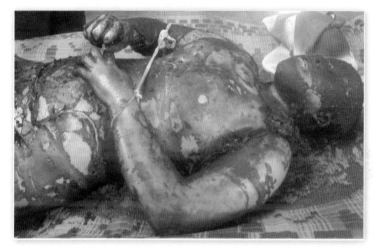

Figure 32 Extensively charred body with pugilistic attitude

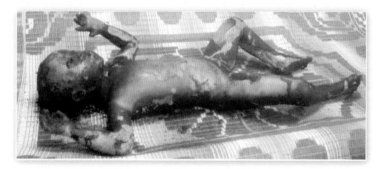

Figure 33 Boxer's attitude in a charred body of a child

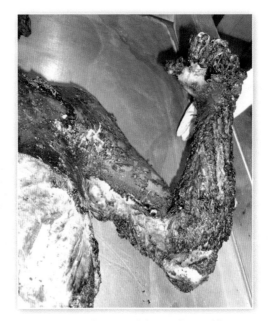

Figure 34 Extensive burns with heat splits and flexion attitude

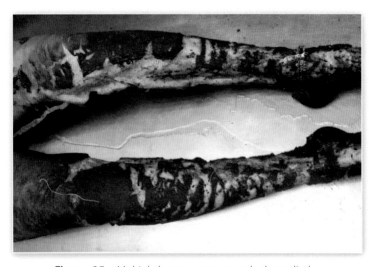

Figure 35 Multiple heat ruptures over the lower limbs

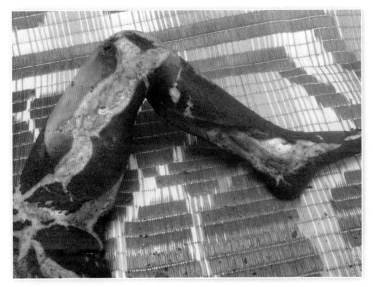

Figure 36 Heat lacerations over the inner aspect of lower limb

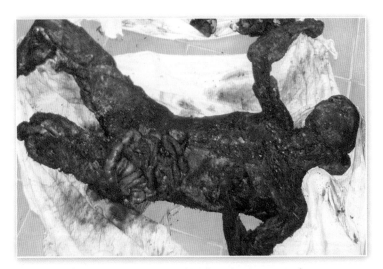

Figure 37 Extensively charred body with protrusion of intestines

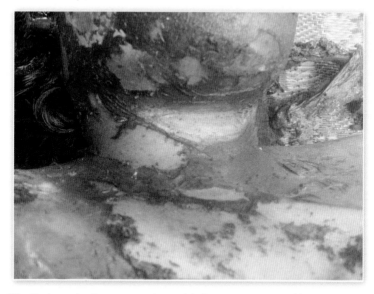

Figure 38   Horizontal pale area over the neck in burn injuries resembling strangulation mark

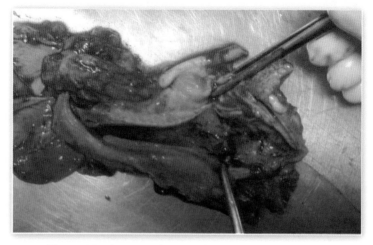

Figure 39   Soot particles in trachea in antemortem burns

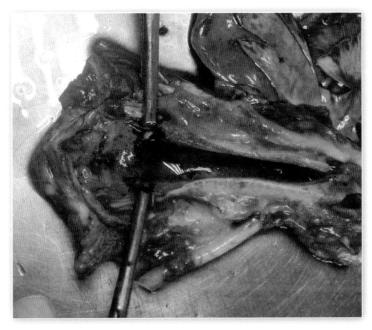

Figure 40   Airways showing soot particles and petechial hemorrhages in antemortem burns

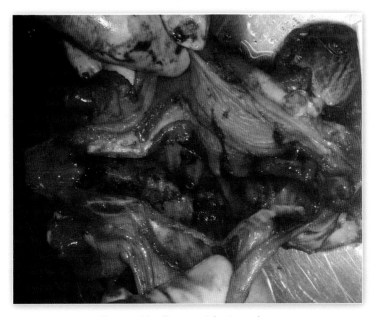

Figure 41   Soot particles in trachea

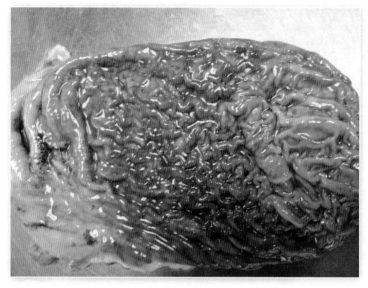

Figure 42   Congested gastric mucosa and presence of soot particles in the stomach

CHAPTER 4

Electrical Injuries

Electrical injuries are caused due to the contact of human body with electric current. Consequently the electric current passes through the body causing deleterious effects. The specific diagnostic sign of electrocution is the electric mark or the Joule burn. This usually appear as crater, round to oval in shape and sometimes associated with charring. Sometimes the mark may have a pattern similar to the shape of the conductor. High tension electric currents may be associated with burns and charring of the involved body parts. Exit marks vary in shapes and sizes and are similar to entry wounds in appearance. In fatal cases, death usually occurs from cardiac arrhythmias. Manner of death in most cases of electrocution is accidental. Rare cases of suicidal electrocution have also been reported in literature.

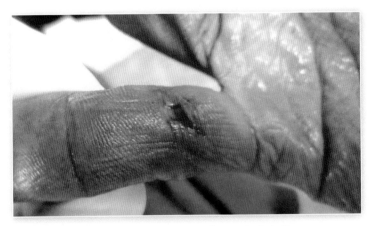

Figure 1 Electrical entry mark over the little finger

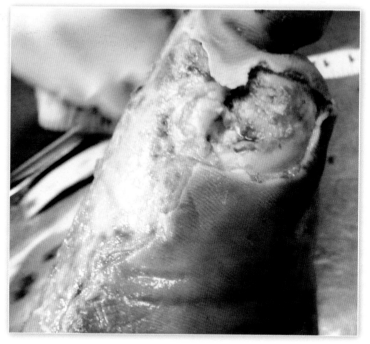

Figure 2 Entry marks in high tension electric current

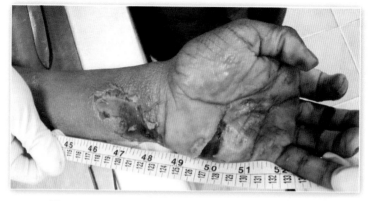

Figure 3 Multiple burns in high tension electric current

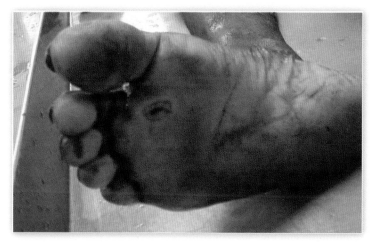

Figure 4   Multiple electric exit wounds on the plantar aspect of foot

CHAPTER 5

Firearm Injuries

Fire arms are classified as rifled and smooth-bored weapons.

Appearance of the injuries sustained by the firearms depends primarily on the type of weapon used, nature of ammunition and the range of firing.

Injuries caused by firearms are characterized by *Entry* and *Exit* wounds. In injuries caused by rifled firearms, the entry wound is usually smaller than the size of the bullet causing it and is characterized by inverted edges and presence of abrasion and grease collar around the wound. Burning, blackening and tattooing may also be present around the wound and on clothes. Exit wound is larger in size and is characterized by everted margins. Wounds produced by shotguns are not frequently associated with exit wounds. Entry wounds on the internal organs show similar characteristics as the external entry wound with absence of burning, blackening and tattooing.

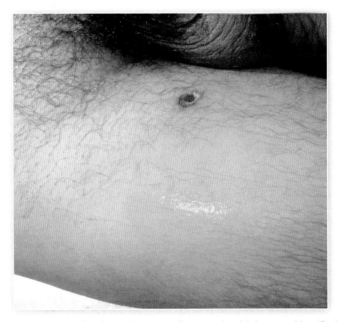

Figure 1 Entry wound with an abrasion collar over the thigh caused by rifled firearm

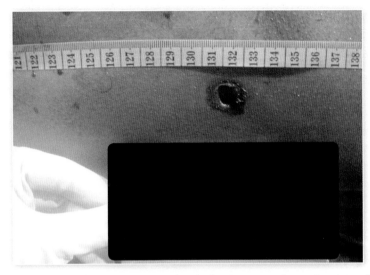

Figure 2   Rifled firearm entry wound with abrasion, contusion and grease collar

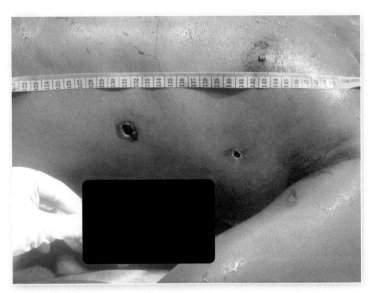

Figure 3   Multiple rifled firearm entry wounds over chest with bullet graze over inner aspect of left arm

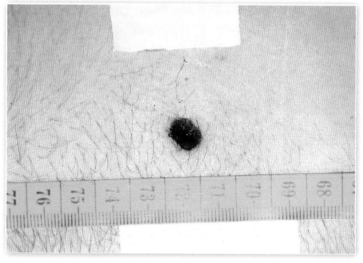

Figure 4   Rifled firearm entry wound depicting the direction of firing

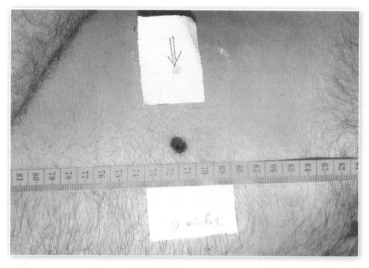

Figure 5   Rifled firearm entry wound

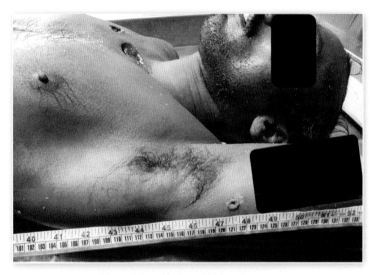

Figure 6 Rifled firearm exit wound on the inner aspect of left arm

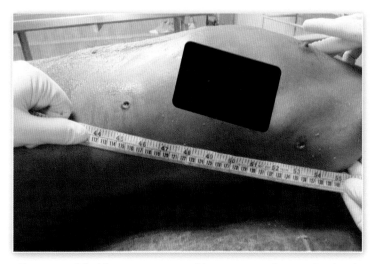

Figure 7 Rifled firearm entry wound (outer aspect of upper chest) and exit wound (left abdominal flank)

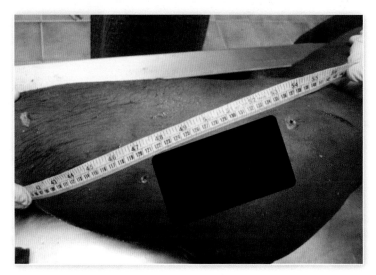

Figure 8   Multiple rifled firearm entry wounds

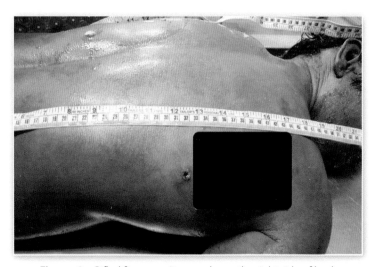

Figure 9   Rifled firearm exit wound over the right side of back

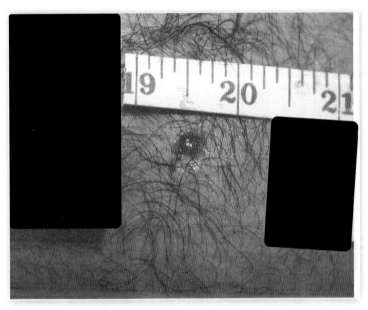

Figure 10   Exit wound caused by rifled firearm

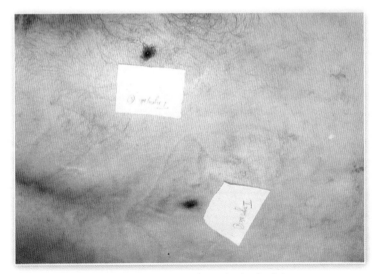

Figure 11   Entry wounds on the back of chest

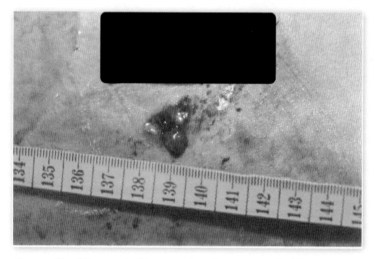

Figure 12 Exit wound with protrusion of tissues in a rifled firearm injury

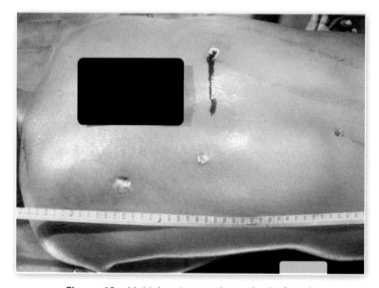

Figure 13 Multiple exit wounds over back of trunk

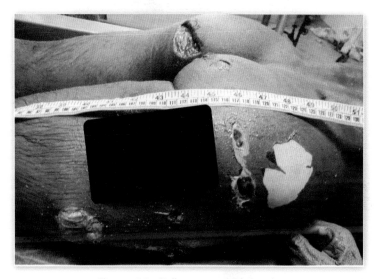

Figure 14   Bullet graze over buttocks

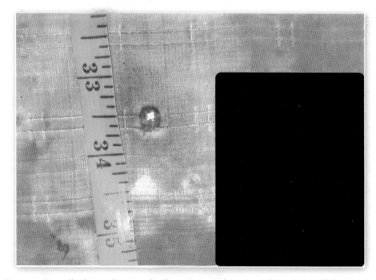

Figure 15   Clothing showing bullet entry and surrounding areas of blackening

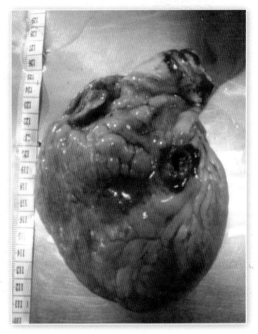

Figure 16   Rifled firearm entry wound with contused
margins over the heart

CHAPTER 6

Regional Injuries

REGIONAL INJURIES

Injuries and death due to trauma are inescapable from the modern way of life. Injuries to the head are very frequent secondary to traffic accidents, assaults and falls.

- **Closed head injury:** In a traumatic episode, if the dura remains intact, it is called closed head injury irrespective of whether the skull is fractured or not.
- **Open head injury:** In a traumatic episode, if the dura is lacerated or torn, it is called an open head injury as it is open to possible infection.

Scalp

A contusion over the scalp, well covered with hair, is better appreciated by palpation than inspection. An effusion of blood over the forehead may gravitate (Indirect trauma) down to the loose tissue causing black eyes. Injuries to scalp predispose the victim to intracranial infections through diploic veins.

Skull

The adult skull is a remarkably strong structure. It is not resilient and tends to fracture if subjected to undue stress. The varieties of fractures seen in medicolegal autopsies are—fissure, stellate, depressed, elevated, gutter comminuted and ring fracture. The fracture may involve the vault or base or both. The base of the skull is relatively weak, by virtue of its irregular shape and several foramina passing through it and is therefore the most common site of skull fractures. In all medicolegal autopsies, the dura should be stripped from the vault and the base so that the fractures can be better appreciated.

Brain Injuries

Brain injuries are classified according to the main effect of trauma as:
1. Acceleration/deceleration injuries are—Diffuse neuronal injuries, diffuse axonal injuries and subdural hematomas.
2. Impact injuries are—Cerebral concussion, cerebral contusions, cerebral lacerations and intracranial hemorrhages (epidural, subdural, subarachnoid and intracerebral hemorrhages).

Trauma to the Heart

According to Mortiz, the common sites of traumatic rupture of heart are—right atrium, left ventricle, right ventricle, left atrium, interventricular septum and valves. In traumatic rupture, the heart is generally ruptured on the right side and towards its base.

Trauma to the Liver

It is susceptible to injury because of its large size, central location and relative friability. The rupture usually involves the right lobe, the convex surface and the inferior border. Death is due to hemorrhage.

Trauma to the Spleen

Its susceptibility to injury is due to weakness of its supporting tissues, thinness of capsule and extreme friability of pulp. The rupture usually involves the concave surface. Death is due to profuse hemorrhage.

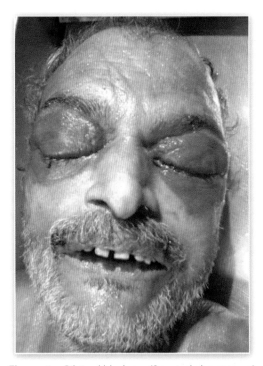

Figure 1   Bilateral black eye (Spectacle hematoma)

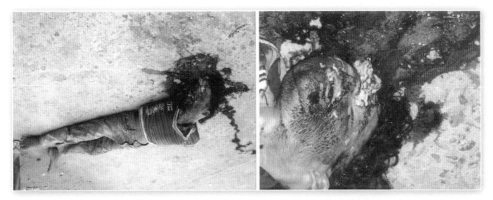

Figure 2   Crushed head with protrusion of brain substance at the scene of vehicular accident

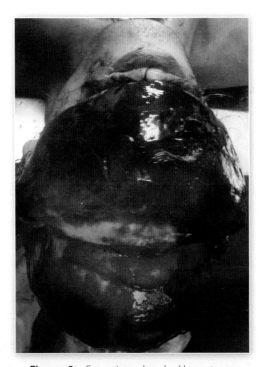

Figure 3   Extensive subscalpal hematoma

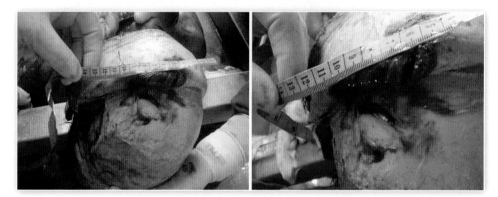

Figure 4   Subscalpal contusion with split laceration

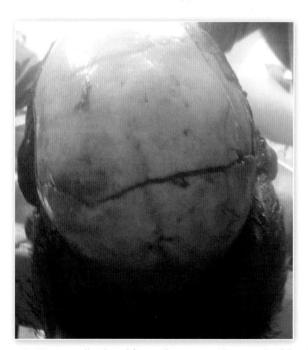

Figure 5   Horizontally placed fissure fracture involving vault of the skull

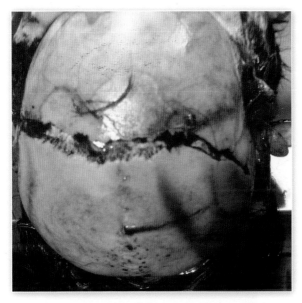

Figure 6   Diastatic (Sutural) fracture involving coronal suture

Depressed comminuted fracture: This is also known as complex fracture. The bone is fractured into fragments due to heavy blunt impact or violent fall. This is as a result of multiple adjacent fissured fractures **(Figs 7 to 9)**.

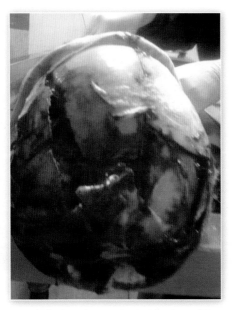

Figure 7   Depressed displaced comminuted fracture of the vault of the skull

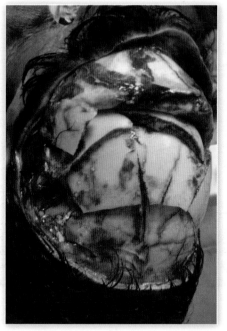

Figure 8   Depressed comminuted fracture of the vault with overriding of cranial bones

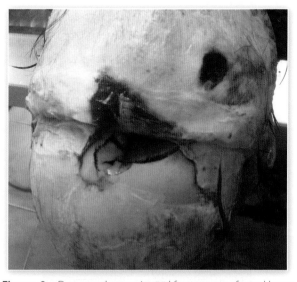

Figure 9   Depressed comminuted fracture over frontal bone

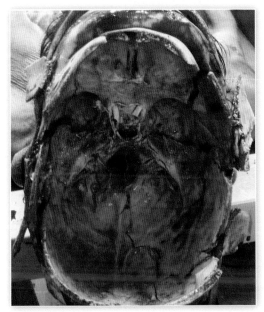

Figure 10   Hinge fracture involving the middle cranial fossa

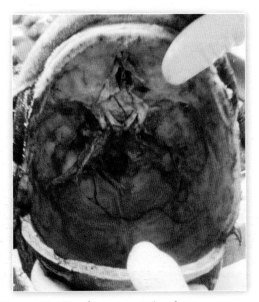

Figure 11   Ring fracture encircling foramen magnum

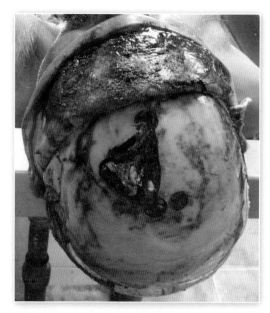

Figure 12   Multiple circular burr hole (Craniotomy wound) over
left frontoparietal region

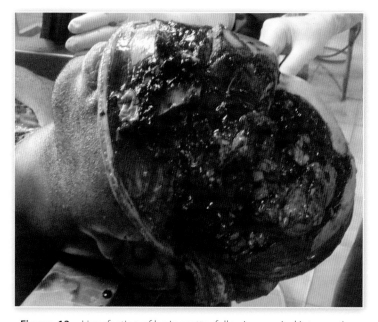

Figure 13   Liquefaction of brain matter following surgical intervention

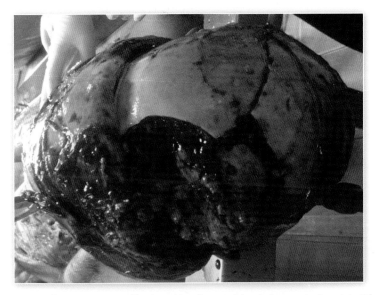

Figure 14   Liquefactive necrosis of brain with adherent blood clots and missed skull fragments

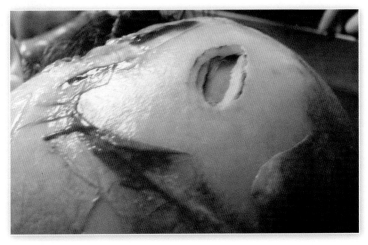

Figure 15   Depressed fracture (Signature fracture) involving
outer table of the skull

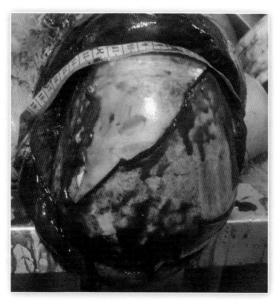

Figure 16 Obliquely placed fissure fracture involving vault of skull

Burst fracture: When the force of impact over the skull is great, the broken pieces of bone get displaced **(Figs 17 to 20)**.

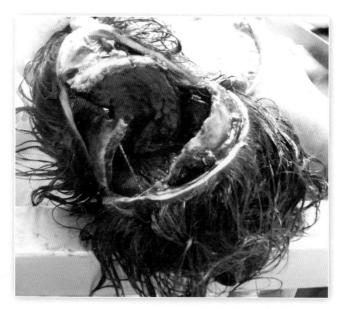

Figure 17 Burst fracture of the skull with displaced skull fragments

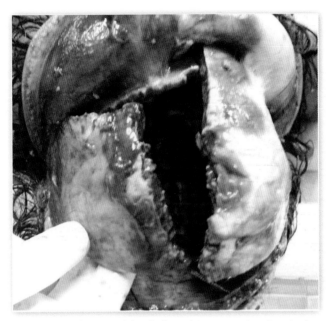

Figure 18 Burst fracture of the skull involving coronal and sagittal sutures

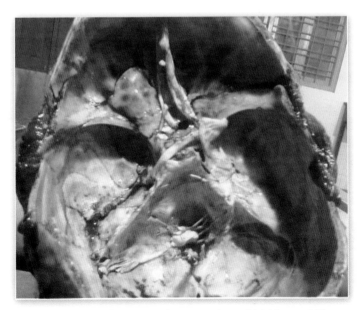

Figure 19 Burst fracture involving anterior and middle cranial fossa

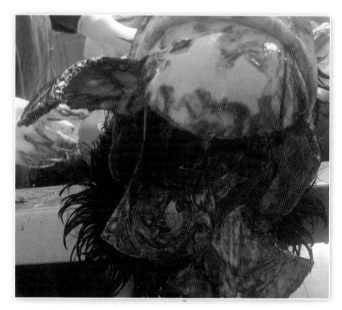

Figure 20   Burst fracture involving vault and base of cranium

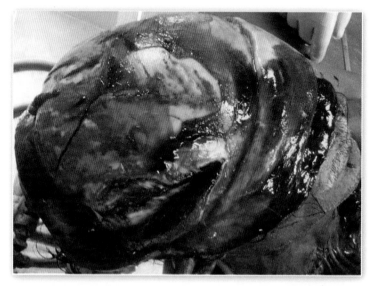

Figure 21   Linear fracture extending to coronal suture (Diastatic fracture)

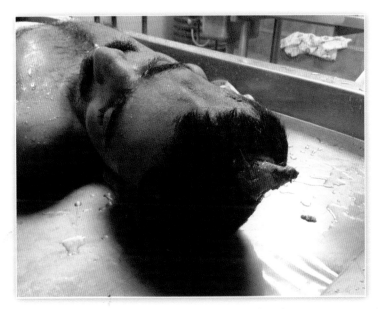

Figure 22 Protrusion of fractured skull fragment through scalp in a run over accident

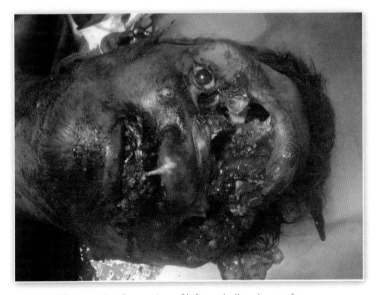

Figure 23 Excavation of left eye ball and root of nose

Pontine hemorrhage is a type of intracranial hemorrhage where bleeding occurs in the pontine region which could be spontaneous or traumatic **(Figs 24 to 26)**.

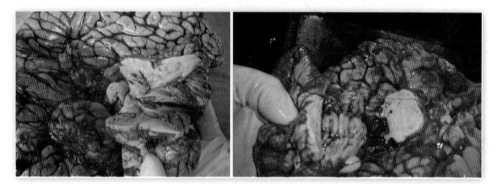

Figure 24 Pontine hemorrhage

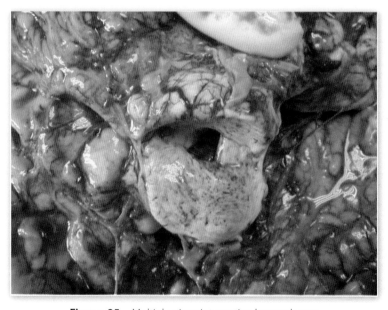

Figure 25 Multiple pinpoint pontine hemorrhages

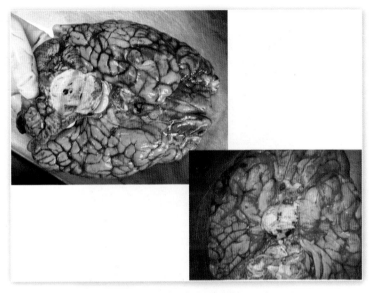

Figure 26   Localized pontine hemorrhage

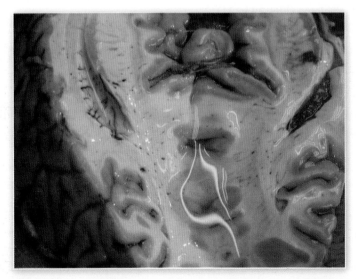

Figure 27   Multiple pinpoint petechial hemorrhages over white matter
suggestive of cerebral hypoxia

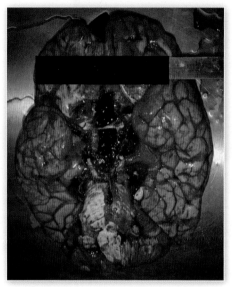

Figure 28   Spontaneous subarachnoid hemorrhage secondary to
rupture of congenital berry aneurysm

Cut section of the brain showing lacerated, contused, necrosed thalamus and basal ganglia with
intraventricular hematoma **(Figs 29 to 31)**.

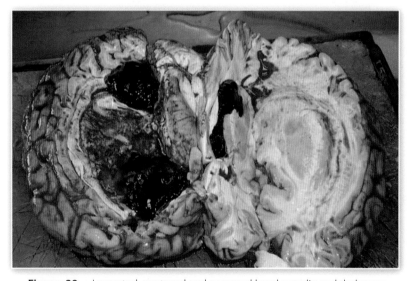

Figure 29   Lacerated, contused and necrosed basal ganglia and thalamus

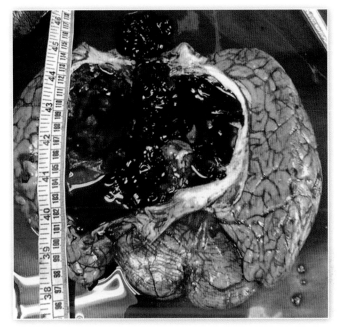

Figure 30   Intraventricular blood clot

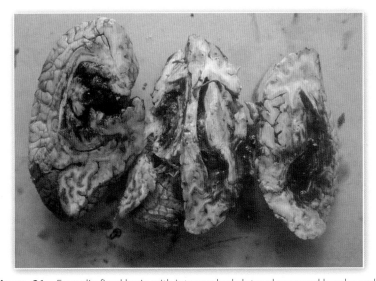

Figure 31   Formalin fixed brain with intracerebral clot and necrosed basal ganglia

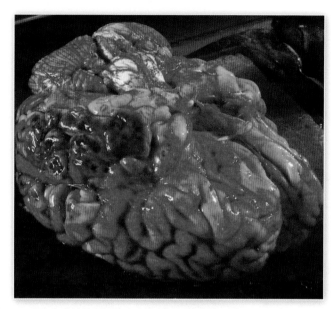

Figure 32   Left temporal lobe contusions with subarachnoid hemorrhage

Multiple pinpoint capillary hemorrhages involving the brain substance: The spontaneous intracerebral hemorrhage is usually seen in internal capsule, basal ganglia, cerebellum, pons, etc. The most common cause is cerebral arteriosclerosis complicated by hypertension. Traumatic hemorrhage is often petechial in nature. It will be often associated with evidence of other injuries such as fracture of skull and contusion of brain **(Figs 33 and 34)**.

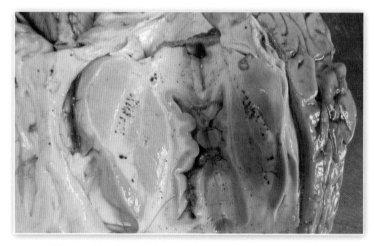

Figure 33   Petechial hemorrhages over internal capsule

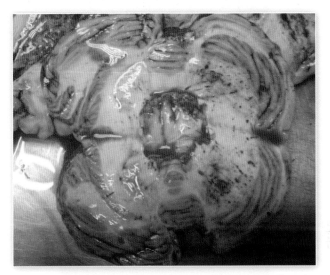

Figure 34 Multiple pinpoint hemorrhages involving cerebellar substance

Extradural hemorrhage occurs outside the dura mater and the clots formed exert pressure over the brain. The source of bleeding is mainly from the meningeal vessels and are often associated with skull fractures **(Figs 35 to 37)**.

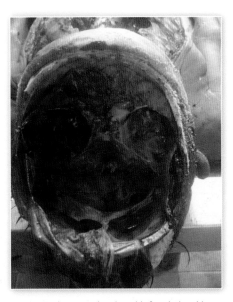

Figure 35 Right extradural and left subdural hematoma

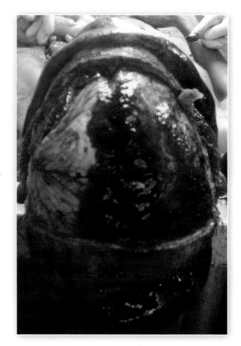

Figure 36 Midline extradural clot

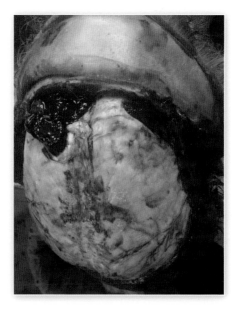

Figure 37 Left frontal extradural hematoma

Subdural hemorrhage occurs between dura and arachnoid mater. It usually appears as a diffuse blood film or clot. The source of bleeding are the dural sinuses, communicating veins, etc. Extensive subdural hematoma can cause death due to cerebral compression **(Figs 38 to 41)**.

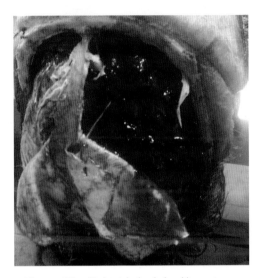

Figure 38   Right sided subdural hematoma

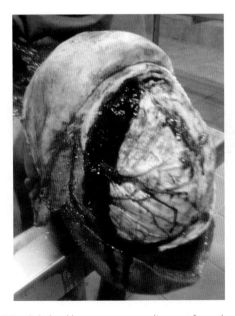

Figure 39   Subdural hematoma extruding out from the cut dura

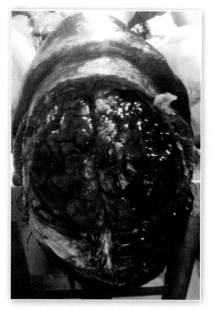

Figure 40   Right sided subdural hematoma and diffuse subarachnoid hemorrhage

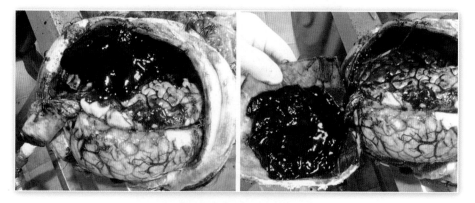

Figure 41   Subdural hematoma with compressed ipsilateral cerebral hemisphere

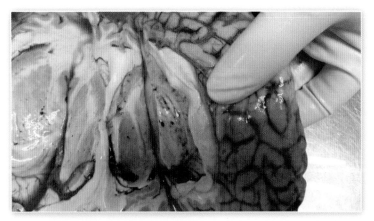

Figure 42 Petechial hemorrhages involving basal ganglia

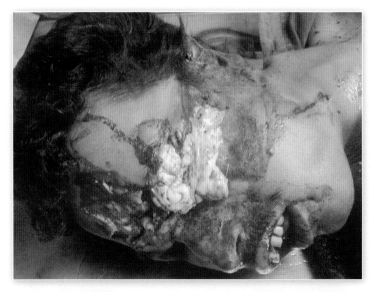

Figure 43 Gross flattening of left side of the face with protruded brain
mater due to run over by a heavy vehicle

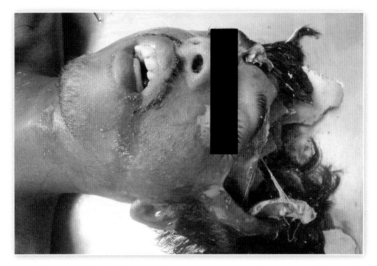

Figure 44   Burst fracture of the skull secondary to traumatic crush injury with loss of brain substance

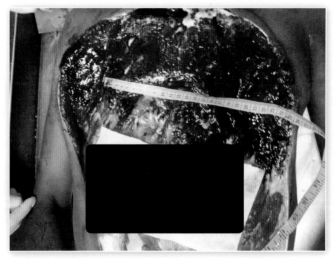

Figure 45   Diffuse contusions over front of chest on reflection of skin

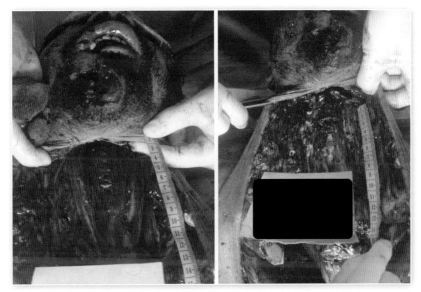

Figure 46   Fracture-dislocation of cervical vertebra (C3–C4)

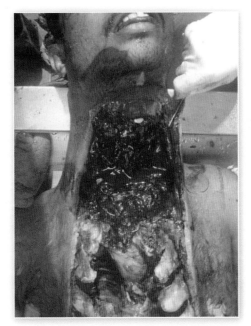

Figure 47   Missing cervical segment (C3–C6) secondary to crush injury to neck in a railway mishap

During fall from height, when the person lands on both feet or buttock the force will be transmitted to the leg bones, hip, vertebral column and to the skull, resulting in fracture-dislocation of vertebral column **(Figs 48 and 49)**.

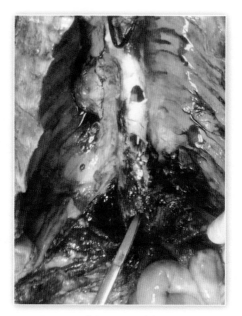

Figure 48 Fracture-dislocation of thoracolumbar vertebra

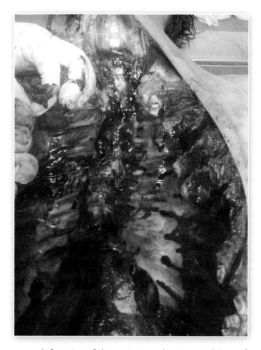

Figure 49 Curvature deformity of thoracic vertebra secondary to fracture-dislocation

Blunt impacts to abdomen need not always produce external injuries, as the abdomen is yielding and the force will be dissipated internally injuring the internal organs **(Figs 50 to 54)**.

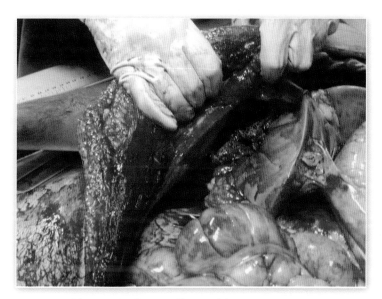

Figure 50   Ruptured liver with hemoperitoneum

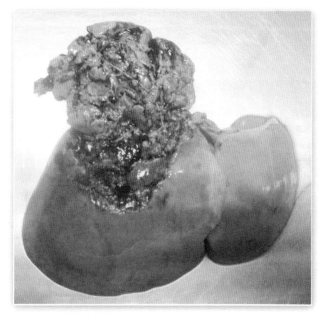

Figure 51   Rupture of anterior and superior surface of right lobe of liver

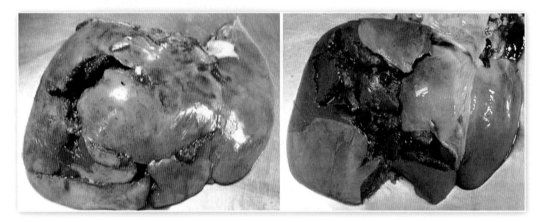

Figure 52   Transparenchymal lacerations of right lobe of liver

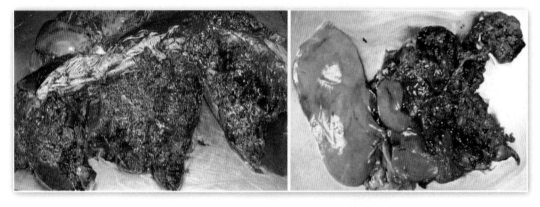

Figure 53   Rupture of liver in a run over accident

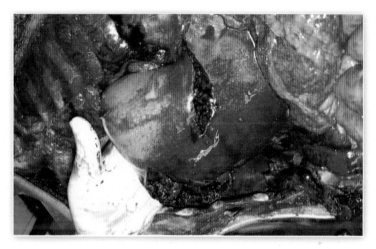

Figure 54 Subcapsular and Transparenchymal laceration of liver

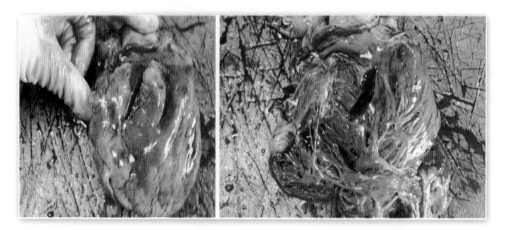

Figure 55 Stab injury over right ventricle due to light pointed sharp weapon

Blunt impacts to the chest can cause abrasions, contusions and lacerations to the chest wall, fractures of the ribs and sternum, contusions and laceration of the lung and heart **(Figs 56 to 62)**.

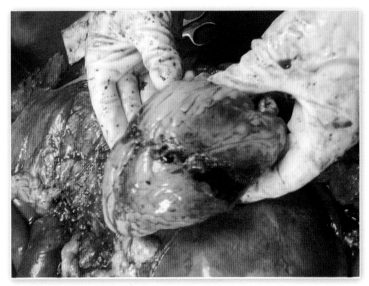

Figure 56 Laceration of left ventricle secondary to bullet injury

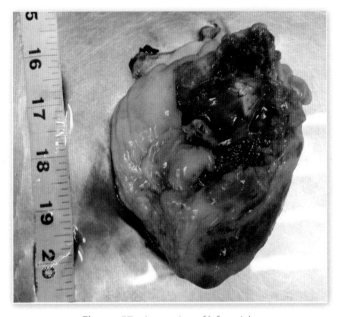

Figure 57 Laceration of left auricle

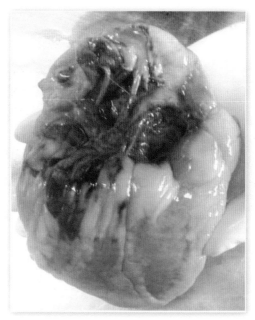

Figure 58   Laceration of right and left auricle with epicardial contusions

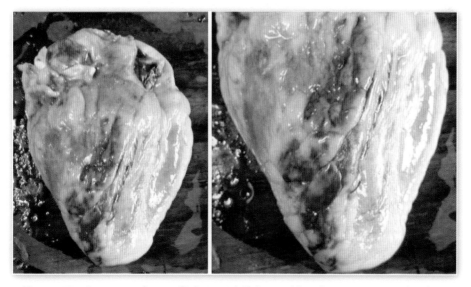

Figure 59   Contusion of apex of left ventricle following blunt force impact over the chest

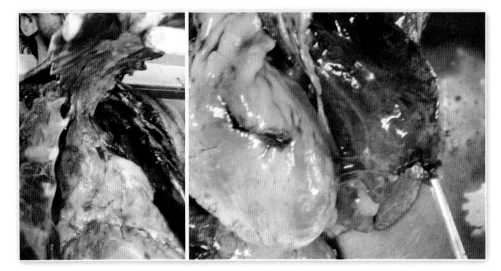

Figure 60   Stab injury to heart and left lung

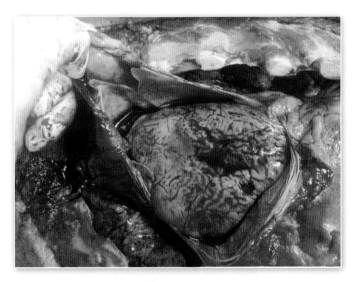

Figure 61   Demonstration of hemopericardium by opening the pericardial sac

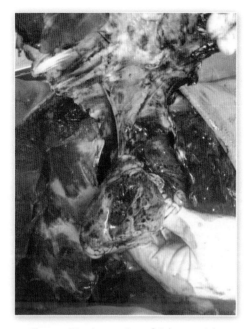

Figure 62 Laceration of right ventricle

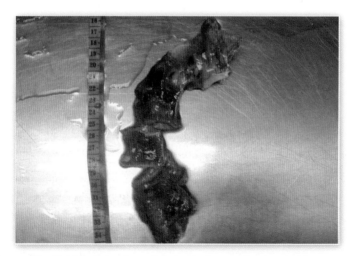

Figure 63 Multiple lacerations of abdominal aorta associated with para-aortic contusion in a road traffic accident

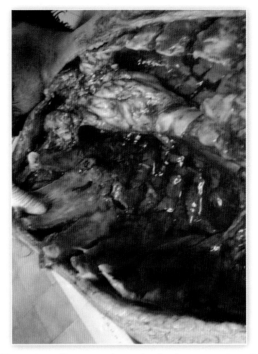

Figure 64   Dissection of intercostal muscles for demonstration of fractured ribs

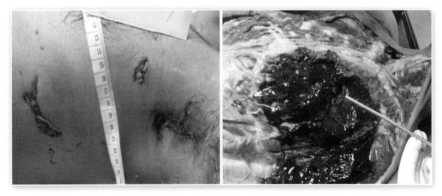

Figure 65   Stab injury over the left side of chest with fracture of 4th rib

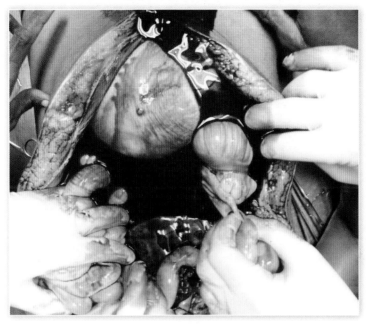

Figure 66 Retroperitoneal hematoma and hemoperitoneum secondary to blunt force impact over lower trunk

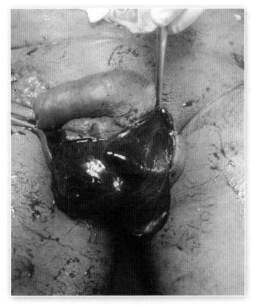

Figure 67 Dissection of the scrotal sac demonstrating hematoma secondary to blunt force trauma

CHAPTER 7

Transportation Injuries

7a   ROAD TRAFFIC ACCIDENTS

Pedestrian Injuries

Three pattern of injuries are seen:
1. **Primary impact injuries** by the vehicle striking the victim.
2. **Secondary impact injuries** due to the victim falling over the offending vehicle after the primary impact.
3. **Secondary injuries** due to the victim falling on the ground or any other object.

Bumper Fracture

Fracture of the tibia and fibula of one or both legs resulting from the impact caused by the projecting part of any vehicle.

Degloving Injuries

When a limb is run over by the wheel of a vehicle, the skin and subcutaneous fat may be dragged away from the deeper muscles with or without any break in the continuity of the skin, resulting in degloving injuries.

Pattern of Injuries to the Driver and Occupants of a Motor Vehicle

In motors car accidents, the injuries may vary depending on the position of the occupants. The unrestrained driver in frontal impact injuries can sustain lacerations to liver, lungs, heart and aorta due to steering wheel impact. The driver can sustain "Whiplash injuries" due to sudden hyperflexion followed by rebound hyperextension of the neck. The unrestrained front seat occupant and the driver are commonly ejected out of the windscreen [Ejection crash injuries] sustaining fractures of the skull and cerebral injuries. In forceful deceleration impact, the unrestrained rear seat occupants are either projected forwards or ejected out from the windscreen sustaining head injuries.

Dicing injuries (sparrow feet lacerations): Multiple punctate lacerations of the face are produced due to shattering of the windscreen glass into multiple small fragments with relatively blunt edges. They are relatively superficial **(Figs 1 to 3)**.

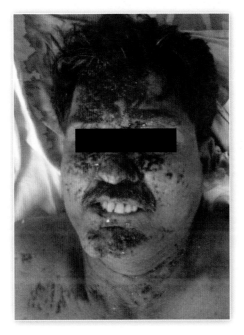

Figure 1   Multiple superficial lacerations over front of face due to windshield impact

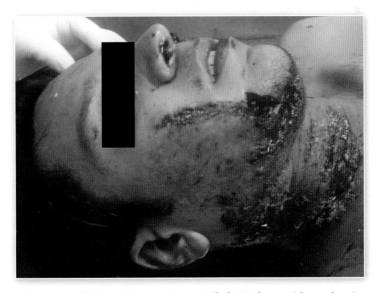

Figure 2   Dicing injuries over lower half of right face and front of neck

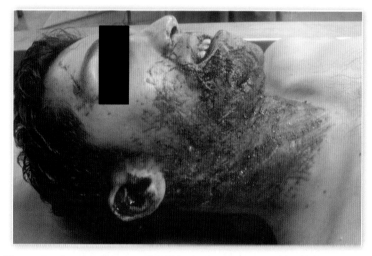

Figure 3   Sparrow feet superficial lacerations due to windshield glass impact

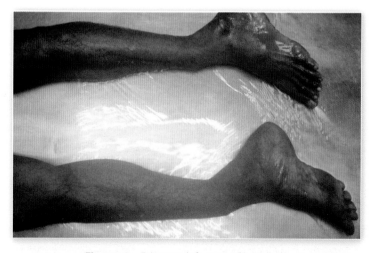

Figure 4   Fracture-deformity of both legs

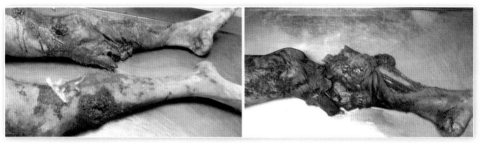

Figure 5 Crush- avulsed laceration secondary to run over by a heavy vehicle

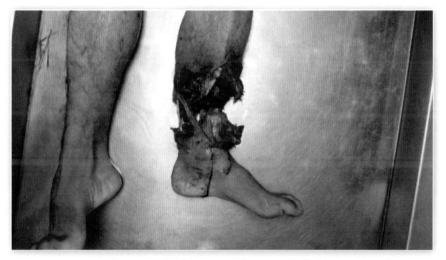

Figure 6 Crush- fracture of lower end of left leg

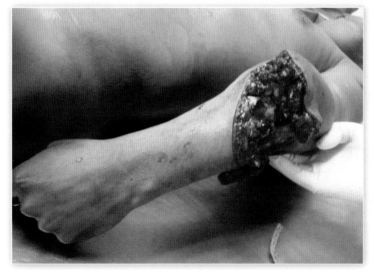

Figure 7 Cut fracture exposing fractured ends of radius and ulna

7b   RAILWAY MISHAPS

Railway injuries are commonly accidental or suicidal, rarely homicidal in nature. The bodies recovered from the railway mishap is always a big dilemma to the autopsy surgeon as to differentiate between antemortem and postmortem injuries, since the death is instantaneous in run over cases and the vital reaction will be minimal. The victim will be hit by a speeding train while crossing or walking along the railway line or jumping in front of it. During the impact, the victim will be thrown forward and sometimes run over. In such cases, the injuries sustained will be of a dismembering nature. It may be difficult to give any opinion if the body is decomposed or badly crushed and mutilated.

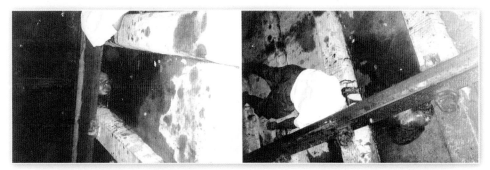

Figure 1   Crime scene of a railway mishap—a case of suicidal decapitation

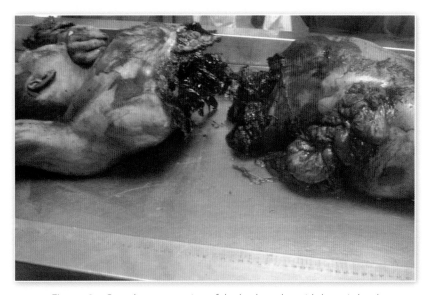

Figure 2   Complete transection of the body at the mid-thoracic level

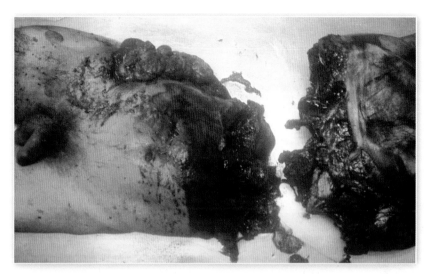

Figure 3   Complete transection of the body at the mid-thoracic level exposing crushed/greased muscles and underlying transected vertebral column

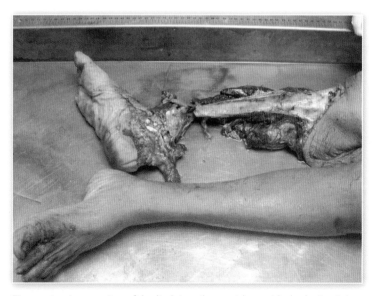

Figure 4   Amputation of the limb in railway mishap with degloving injury

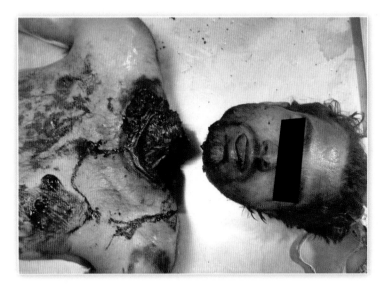

Figure 5   Decapitation in a case of railway runover accident

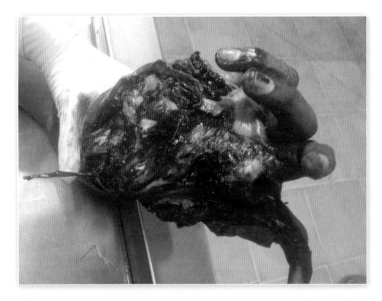

Figure 6   Traumatic crushed hand with exposed underlying multiple fracture of carpal bones

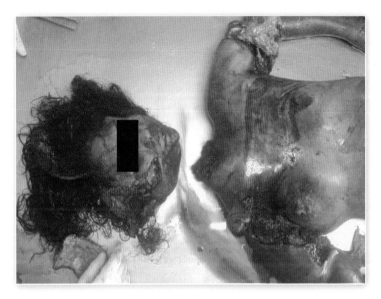

Figure 7   Decapitation injury associated with gross flattening of the chest surface

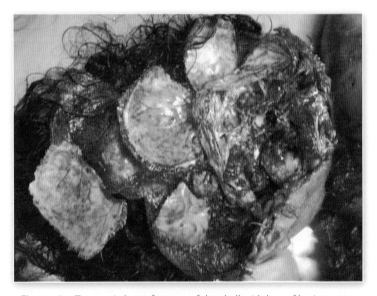

Figure 8   Traumatic burst fracture of the skull with loss of brain matter

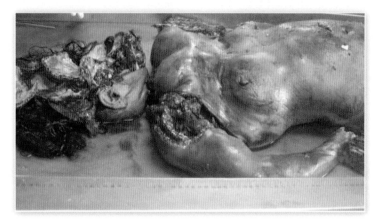

Figure 9   Traumatic crush injury involving head, face and upper half of chest

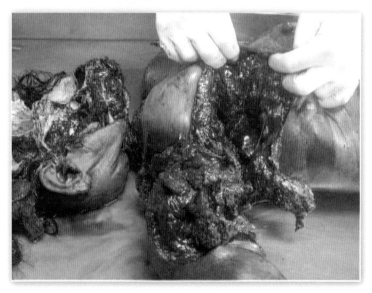

Figure 10   Penetrating injury of the chest due to impact by the projecting part of the railway engine

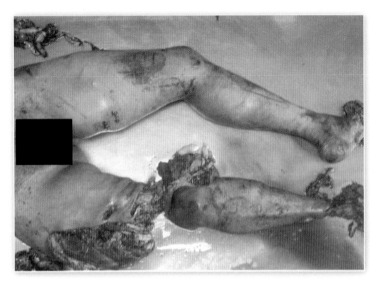

Figure 11   Traumatic amputation of the limb

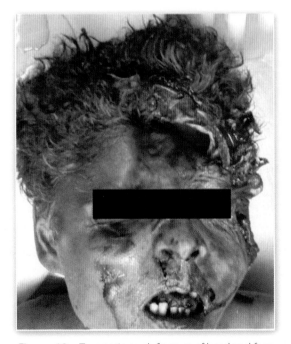

Figure 12   Traumatic crush fracture of head and face

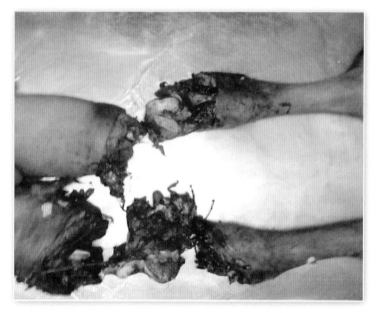

Figure **13**   Traumatic crush amputation of lower limb involving knee joint

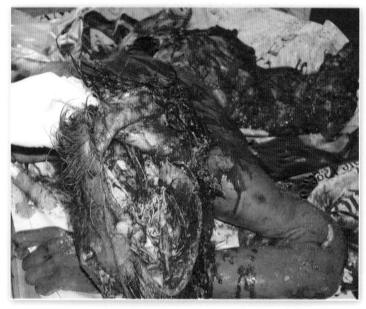

Figure **14**   Crush fracture of the skull exposing the remnants of dura and brain matter

7c AIRCRAFT MISHAPS

Aircraft injuries can occur during the take-off, mid-air flight period, or landing. Injuries sustained in aircraft mishaps may vary accordingly. The injuries can be of acceleration-deceleration type, or smoke inhalation, and burn injuries. Bodies may be extensively burnt and charred if the aircraft catches fire. The primary aim of autopsy in such cases is to establish the identity of the charred remains.

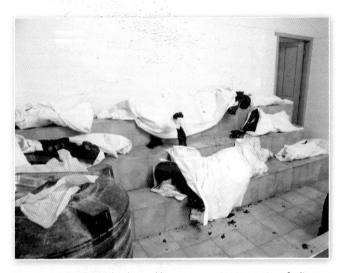

Figure 1 Extensively charred human remains in an aircraft disaster

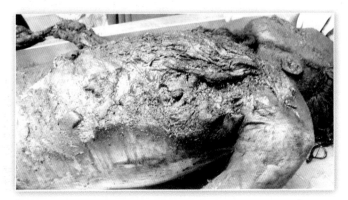

Figure 2 Charred body with multiple postmortem splits

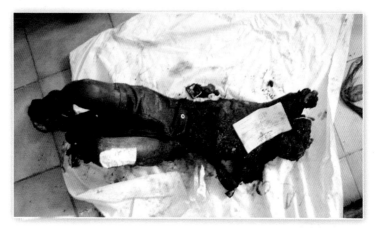

Figure 3 Dismembered charred remains of a child

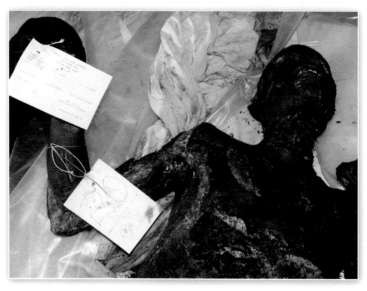

Figure 4 Extensively charred body in pugilistic attitude with multiple postmortem lacerations

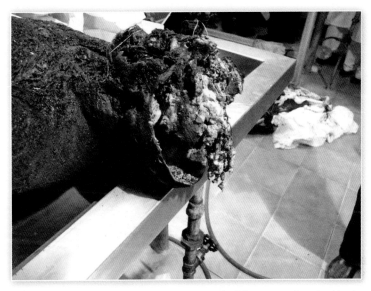

Figure 5   Charred body with postmortem skull fracturs and cooked brain

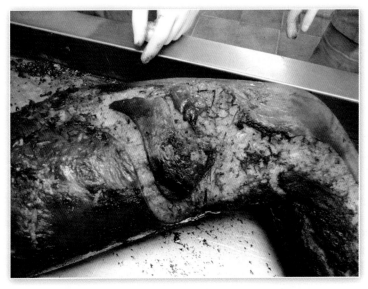

Figure 6   Postmortem splits due to extensive burns

CHAPTER 8

Mechanical Asphyxia

Asphyxia in common parlance means 'lack of oxygen', but etymologically it means 'absence of pulse'.

Mechanical asphyxia results from any mechanical impediment to the airways or restriction of thoracoabdominal movements. Mechanical asphyxia can be classified into different types based upon the causative agent and location of the obstruction or restriction of entry of the air into the respiratory tract as:

- Pressure upon the exterior of the neck structures: Hanging, strangulation, mugging, etc.
- Obstruction of external air passages: Smothering and gagging
- Obstruction of internal air passages: Choking
- Restriction of respiratory movements of the thorax: Traumatic asphyxia, postural asphyxia
- Submersion deaths.

In complete hanging, the entire body weight acts as the constricting force around the neck, whereas in partial/incomplete hanging only a part of the body weight acts as a constricting force, as some part of the body is in contact with floor or any other object in standing, sitting, kneeling and reclining positions. In typical hanging, the knot of the ligature material will be located at the nape of the neck whereas in atypical hanging the knot will be located anywhere around the neck other than the nape **(Figs 1 to 10)**.

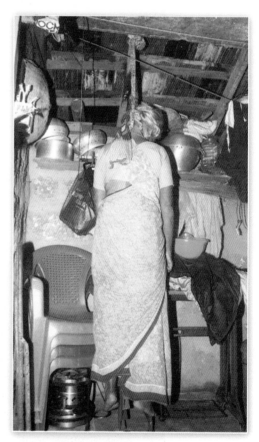

Figure 1 Complete typical hanging with the knot located on the nape of neck

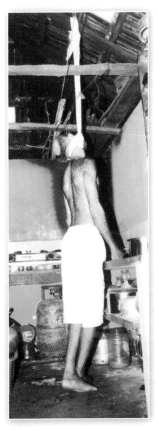

Figure 2 Incomplete atypical hanging with the knot located on the right side of neck

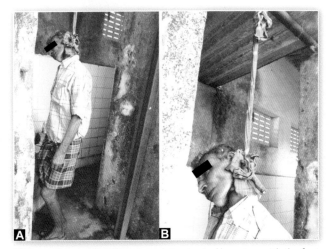

Figures 3A and B (A) Incomplete atypical hanging with the feet touching the ground and the knot located on the right side of neck, (B) Close-up view showing the position of knot

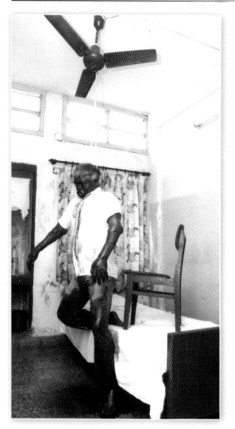

Figure 4 Incomplete atypical hanging with the right upper limb resting on a cot and the knot located on the nape of neck

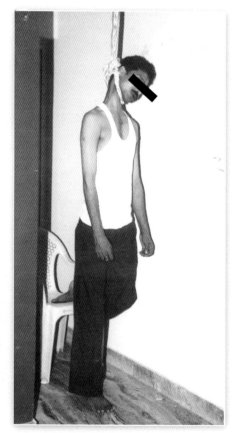

Figure 5 Incomplete atypical hanging with the left foot resting on a chair and the knot located on the right side of neck

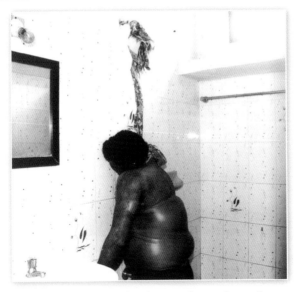

Figure 6   A case of incomplete hanging from a shower faucet with
early signs of decomposition

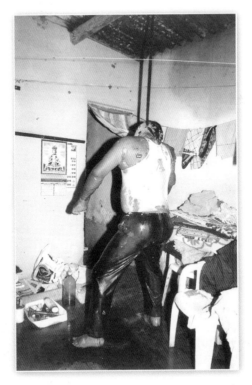

Figure 7   A case of incomplete hanging with
evidence of postmortem blisters and purging

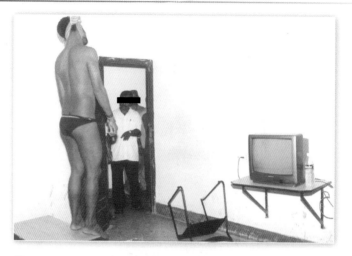

Figure 8 A case of incomplete atypical hanging with the knot on the right side of neck and the feet resting on the table

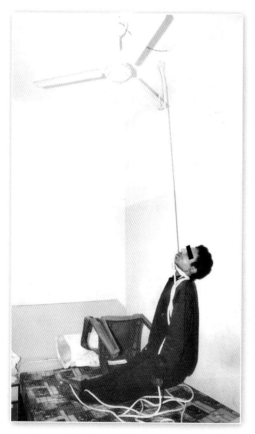

Figure 9 A case of incomplete atypical hanging with multiple loops around the neck

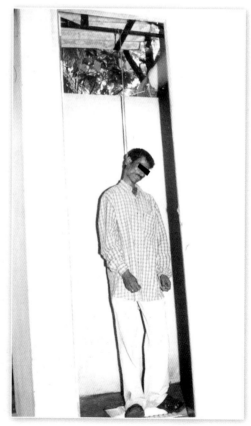

Figure 10 Incomplete atypical hanging with the feet resting on a lavatory pan

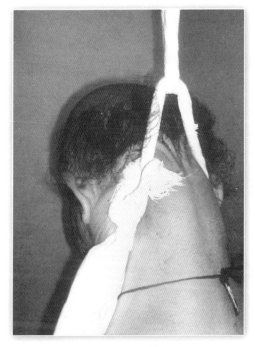

Figure 11   Typical hanging

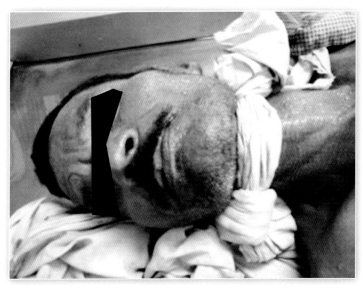

Figure 12   Ligature material with multiple knots

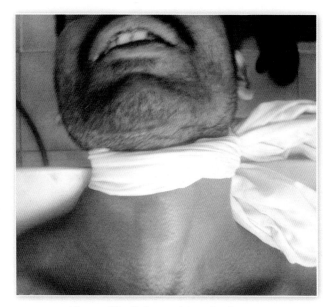

Figure 13   Soft material used as ligature

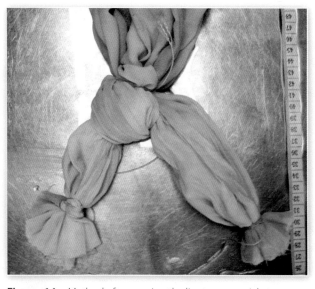

Figure 14   Method of preserving the ligature material at autopsy

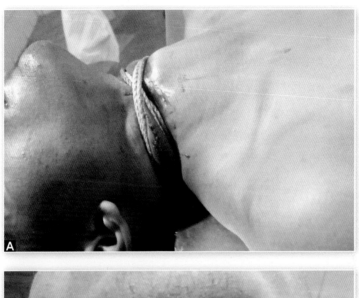

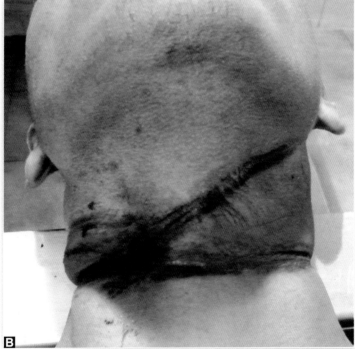

Figures 15A and B   Multiple crisscross patterned grooved abrasions matching the ligature material (nylon rope) around the neck

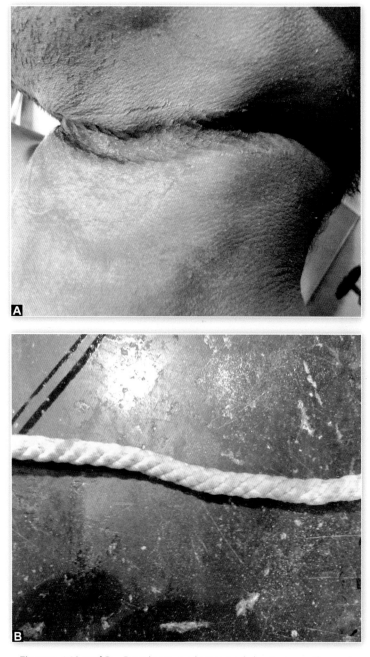

Figures 16A and B   Deeply grooved patterned abrasion over the neck corroborating with the ligature material

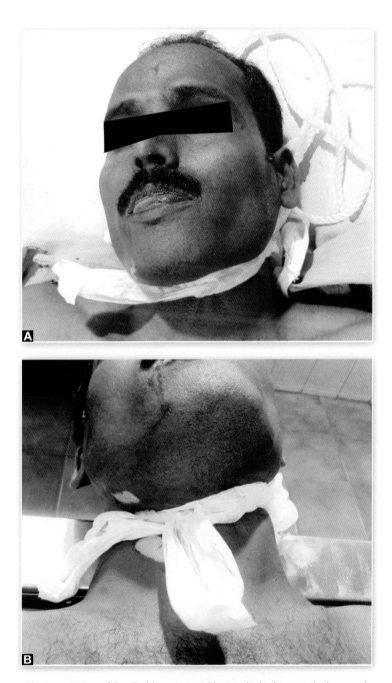

Figures 17A and B   Padding material beneath the ligature (nylon rope)

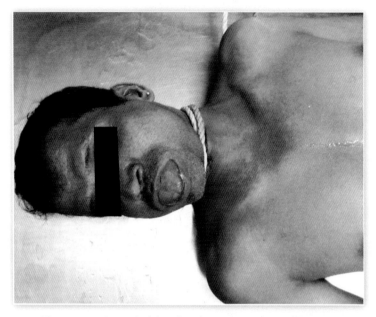

Figure 18   Protruded discolored tongue in a case of hanging

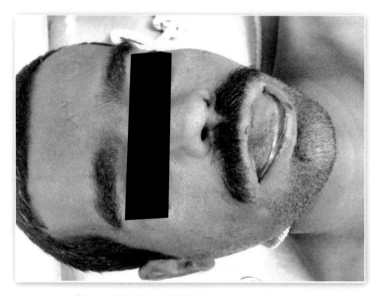

Figure 19   Protruded bitten tongue in hanging

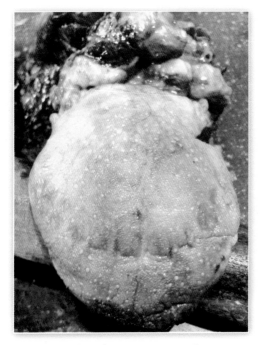

Figure 20   Dental impressions over the tongue

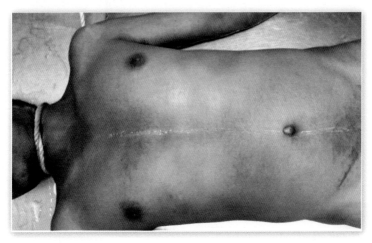

Figure 21   Dried salivary stains over front of the trunk in the midline; a
sign of antemortem hanging

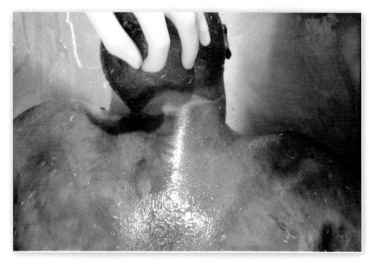

Figure 22   Skin folds of the neck in a decomposed body
simulating ligature mark

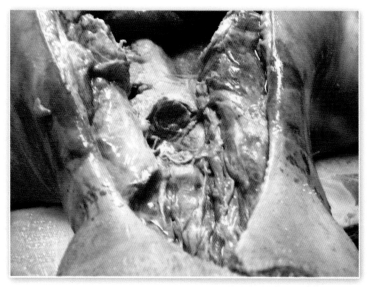

Figure 23   Postmortem displacement of cervical vertebra due to prolonged
suspension in a decomposed body

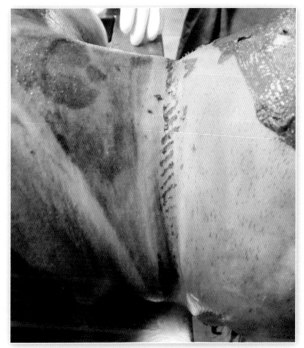

Figure 24 Well-preserved ligature mark in a decomposed body

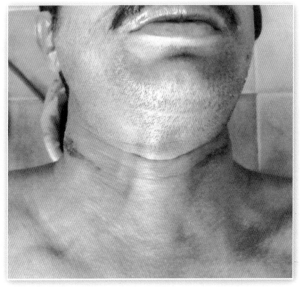

Figure 25 Faint ligature mark on both sides of neck in partial hanging

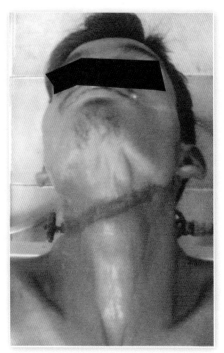

Figure 26   Obliquely placed ligature mark
above the level of thyroid cartilage

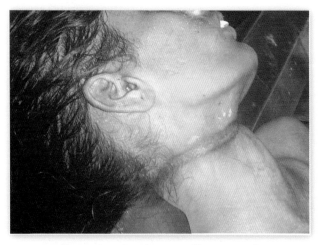

Figure 27   Deeply grooved ligature mark

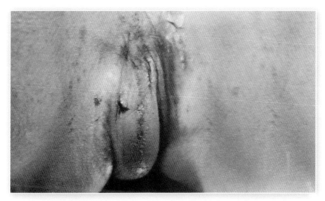

Figure 28 Periligature injuries (rope burns) on neck

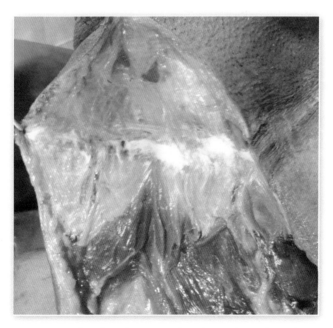

Figure 29 Bloodless dissection of neck revealing white glistening area over the subcutaneous tissue and muscles underneath the ligature mark

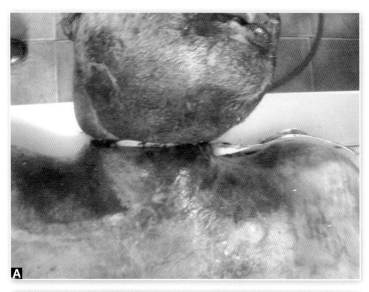

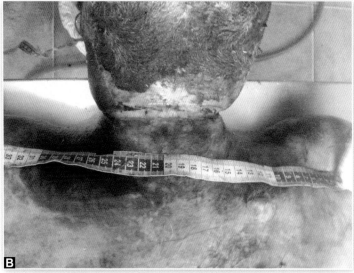

Figures 30A and B   Horizontal mark by a plastic strap in a case of ligature strangulation

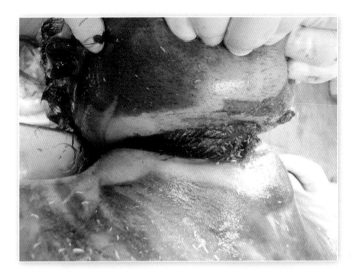

Figure 31 Preserved patterned abrasion (ligature mark) in a decomposed body

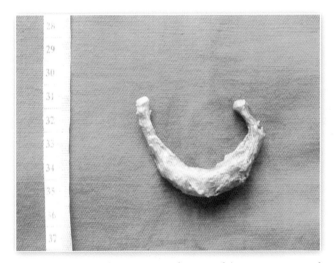

Figure 32 Inward compression fracture of the greater cornu of hyoid bone seen typically in a case of throttling

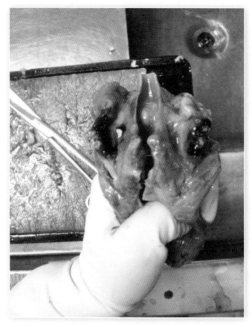

Figure 33 Bilateral fracture of greater cornu of hyoid bone with surrounding contusion in manual strangulation

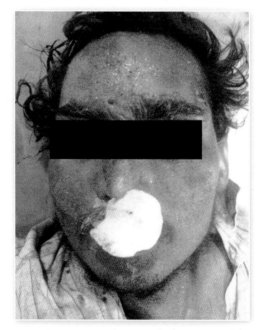

Figure 34 Appearance of copious froth in a case of drowning

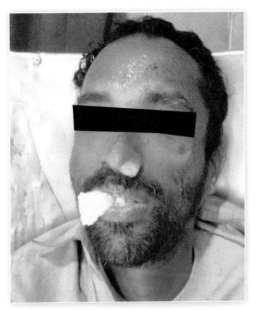

Figures 35 Typical froth (white, copious, fine, lathery, tenacious and persistent) in antemortem drowning

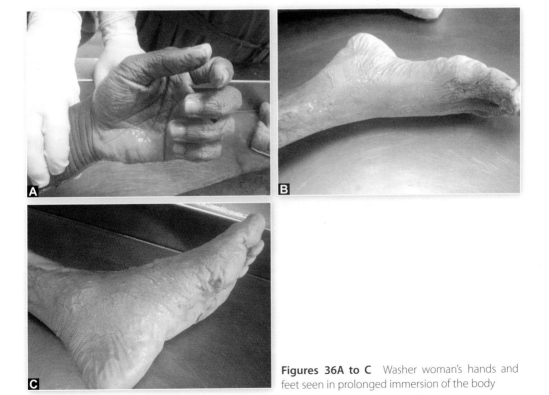

Figures 36A to C Washer woman's hands and feet seen in prolonged immersion of the body

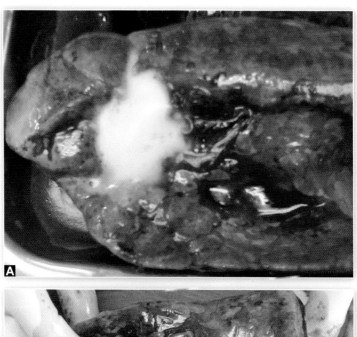

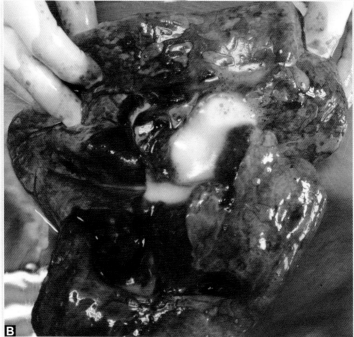

Figures 37A and B Water logged voluminous bulky
lungs with copious froth

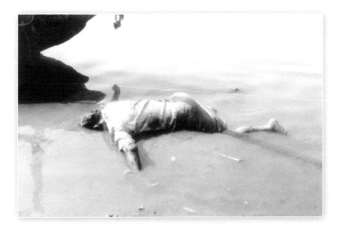

Figure 38   Dead body in a case of drowning being washed ashore

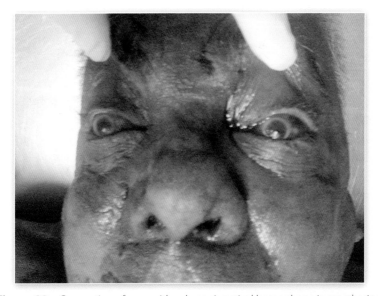

Figure 39   Congestion of eyes with sub-conjunctival hemorrhage in smothering

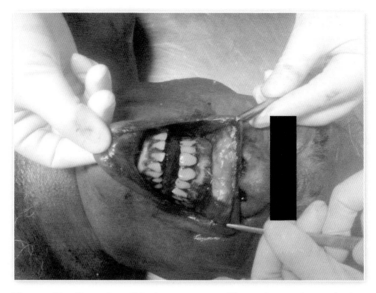

Figure 40 Contusion of the inner aspects of lips and gums in smothering

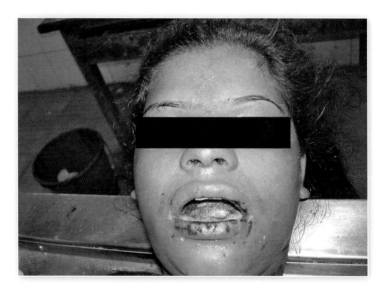

Figure 41 Multiple pressure abrasions over and around the
lips in smothering

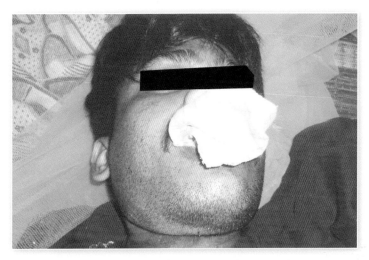

Figure 42   A cloth stuffed into the oral cavity resulting in suffocation (gagging)

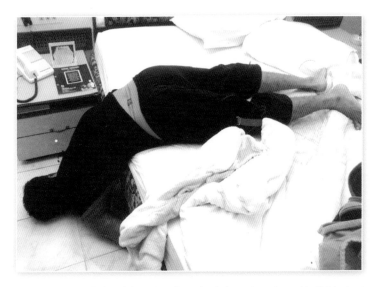

Figure 43   Postural (positional) asphyxia in an intoxicated individual

Index

Page numbers followed by *f* refer to figure